Praise for Jorge Cruise and *8 Minutes in the Morning*

"Jorge Cruise has come up with a great way to jump-start your morning. *8 Minutes in the Morning* is a must for anyone trying to lose weight and get in shape. It works!"

—**Denise Austin,** Host of Lifetime TV's *Daily Workout*

∎

"Jorge shows you how to get great results in less time than it takes to shower in the morning. If you've been procrastinating about starting an exercise program, you have no more excuses."

—**Kathy Smith,** bestselling fitness author

∎

"The number one excuse for not working out is 'Time!' Well, now you have no excuse because Jorge Cruise has the solution for both time and body, *8 Minutes in the Morning*!"

—**Tamilee Webb,** M.A., star of *Buns of Steel* video series

∎

"How great is this program?!? Jorge's is an incredibly easy plan that produces real weight loss and fitness improvements in less than 10 minutes a day, right at home—without gyms, personal trainers, or special foods and supplements. If you want to get fit, firm, and feel better about yourself—even if you've never been successful before—you owe it to yourself to give this program a try!"

—**Catherine Cassidy,** editor-in-chief of *Prevention* magazine

∎

"Hooray for Jorge! At last, a weight-loss expert that explodes misconceptions about fat and introduces how the 'right' fat can make you fit. Hold on for a slimmer and healthier you."

—**Jade Beutler,** author of *Understanding Fats and Oils* and renowned "fat" researcher

"If you can't take 8 minutes out of a 24-hour day to take care of the most important person on this Earth, you are just plain lazy. Jorge will get you up and started."

—**Jack LaLanne,** host of the first nationally syndicated TV exercise show and "The Godfather of Physical Fitness"

■

"Jorge wants to get you super-healthy, not just super-lean."

—**Lisa Klugman,** editor-in-chief of *Fit* magazine

■

"No trips to the gym. No endless walking sessions. No complicated meal plans. A science-based quickie strategy that has already helped millions of folks get slim."

—*Woman's World* magazine

■

"The new program will have you fit, firm and feeling fabulous—no sweat required."

—*First for Women* magazine

■

"The perfect plan when you are short on time."

—*Prevention* magazine

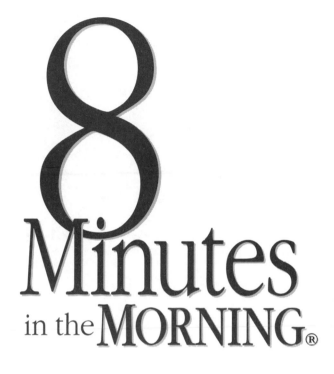

Also by Jorge Cruise

8 Minutos Por La Mañana

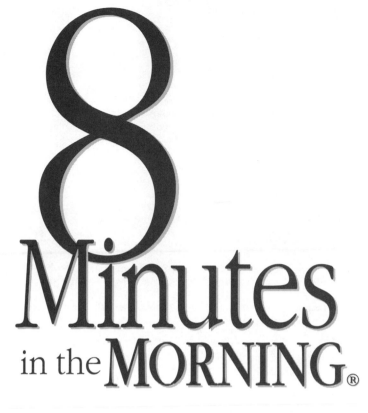

8 Minutes in the MORNING®

A Simple Way to Shed Up to 2 Pounds a Week—GUARANTEED

JORGE CRUISE

The #1 ONLINE WEIGHT-LOSS SPECIALIST
with more than 3 million clients

Foreword by Anthony Robbins, #1 Best-Selling Author

HarperResource
An Imprint of HarperCollins*Publishers*

A hardcover edition of this book was published in 2001 by Rodale.

First HarperResource edition published 2003.

Exercise Photographs © Rodale Inc.
8 Minutes in the Morning is a registered trademark, and *Jorge Cruise* and *Eat Fat to Get Fit* are trademarks of Jorge Cruise, Inc., and may not be used without permission.
Jorge Cruise's athletic gear provided by Adidas, Ulloa, and Crunch Fitness

Cover and Interior Design by: Christopher Rhoads

"Exchange Lists for Meal Planning" © 1995, American Diabetes Association, Inc., and American Dietetic Association. Used with permission.

Library of Congress Cataloging-in-Publication Data

Cruise, Jorge.
    8 minutes in the morning : a simple way to shed up to 2 pounds a week—
guaranteed / Jorge Cruise ; foreword by Anthony Robbins.— 1st [HarperCollins] ed.
      p. cm.
    Previously published: Emmaus, PA : Rodale, 2001.
    Includes index.
    ISBN 0-06-050538-9
    1. Diet.   2. Exercise.   3. Reducing exercises.   4. Health.   5. Weight loss.   I.
Title: Eight minutes in the morning.   II. Title.
    RA781 .C78   2003
    613.7—dc21   2002027302

03 04 05 06 07 08 QW 20 19

To two very special angels—

my mother, Gloria, who is my brilliant star in the sky—

and to Heather, my best friend, wife and soul mate.

Acknowledgments

First, I want to acknowledge the more than 3 million (and growing) cyberspace clients that I have had the privilege to coach. Without their feedback, insight, and support, my 8 Minutes in the Morning program would not be the success it is today.

I must thank Oprah Winfrey, the woman who launched my career. She invited me to be a guest on her show in Chicago and introduced me to two people whose lives had changed because of my weight-loss Web site. I will never forget that day. It was from that moment on that I knew that my Creator had given me a responsibility to take my message and share it with the largest number of people possible.

Heather, my beautiful wife and the most amazing woman I have ever met: Meeting you has changed my life, and I feel so privileged to be sharing this amazing adventure with you. You give my life purpose and juice. All my love, all my life.

Jan Miller, my literary agent, and Michael Broussard, her right hand: Thank you for making the publication of *8 Minutes in the Morning* a reality. I look forward to a lifetime of producing great weight-loss books with you. Also a special thank you to Carolyn Rangel for introducing me to Jan. Thank you, Carolyn, for your faith and friendship.

Rusty Robertson, my marketing mentor: Thank you for your belief in "Jorge" and for your invaluable marketing insights on how to reach the largest number of people possible. You are my model of honesty, integrity, and passion.

Anthony Robbins and Pam Hendrickson, his right hand: Thank you for your friendship, support, and inspiration. Your message is an extraordinary force for good in the world.

My family: To Dad and Grandpa: Thank you for giving me a major boost when I was starting out. To my sister, Marta, for your ongoing love and never-ending support. To my *Abuelita* Maria (grandma) and your lifelong devotion. *Mil besitos.* And of course to my beautiful mama, Gloria, and her many sacrifices that allow me to stand where I am today.

My friends who believed in me: Jason Gregory Smith, Andrew Roorda, Sandi Roorda, Hessel Roorda, Veronique Franccus, Todd Robertson, David Zelcer, Debra Russell, Lisa Druxman, Melissa Johnson, Maggie Barrett, Michael Clark, Dayna Crawford, Valerie Delevante, Jack Williams, the Learning Annex, my Sigma Chi brothers, Laura Ries, Cristina Saralegui, Bruce Barlean, Jade Beutler, Diane Kennedy, Kathy Smith, Dr. Andrew Weil, Jack and Elaine LaLanne, Denise Austin, Tamilee Webb, Arielle Ford, Katherine Kellmeyer, and Arnold Schwarzenegger.

And a special thank-you to: Lisa Sharky, Cathy Chermol, Maryann Bennett, Sandra Aiken, Lisa Katz, my *Good Morning America* military wives, Margaret Breslin Jaqua, Carol Brooks, Ailsa Long, John Monahan, Karen Kraeszig, Adrienne Bergeron, Lisa DelVaglio, Tina Draney, Robert Allen, Kat Carney, Christina Park, all my CNN friends, Cameron Ogletree, Ben Gage, Chuck Verde, Cynthia Davis, all my U.S. Mills friends, Stephanie Tade, Marc Jaffe, Jackie Dornblaser, Neil Wertheimer, Cindy Ratzlaff, Mary Lengle, Abel Delgado, Dana Bacher, Lorraine Rodriguez, Alisa Bauman, Mitch Mandel, Chris Rhodes, Ardie Rodale, Maria Rodale, Steve Murphy, all my Rodale friends, Lyssa Keusch, Megan Newman, Mary Ellen Curley, Shelby Meizlik, Paul Olsewski, Suzie Sisoler, Kate Stark, and all my HarperCollins friends.

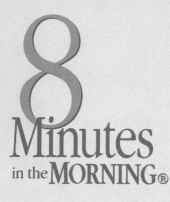

Contents

PART ONE: Jorge and You

Chapter 1

Chapter 2

Chapter 3

PART TWO: How It Works

Chapter 4

Chapter 5

Chapter 6

PART THREE: The Program

You've Got the Power

By Anthony Robbins, author of the #1 bestseller *Awaken the Giant Within*

Congratulations on your commitment to improving the quality of your life! I truly believe that physical health and vitality are the basis for an outstanding life, and I guarantee that when your body is in optimum condition, you will enjoy amazing energy, allowing you to grow, contribute to others, and lead a fulfilling and passionate life. With such energy, your possibilities are limitless. Not only will you feel outstanding physically but also you will have a mental clarity that will enable you to focus on taking control of your future and making your dreams a reality.

Remember: Your body is not your enemy! Many people, in their desire to be superachievers, create immense amounts of stress for themselves. Unfortunately, food becomes the vehicle by which they alleviate that stress, and the result is poor health and often a feeling of discouragement or even desperation.

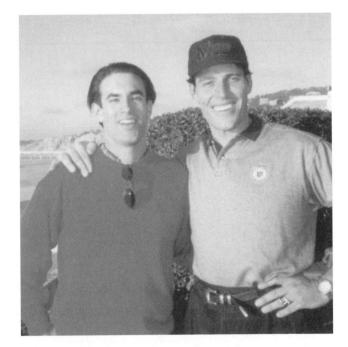

We all know that we should change our habits to improve our lifestyles. What happens is that we make the decision to begin a new health program, but then something else comes up and we don't have time. We quit. The reason we encounter such challenges is because this decision is a "should," not a "must." And as I tell people all the time, we are constantly "shoulding" all over ourselves. Unless our decision becomes a part of who we are—our identity—the changes we make will be only temporary.

Once health becomes a must, there is something else I recommend to help people stay focused: coaching. Working with someone who understands your frustrations and can encourage you in overcoming the challenges along the way will keep you on track and even accelerate the pace at which you achieve your desired results.

Jorge Cruise's *8 Minutes in the Morning* can be that coach. Jorge Cruise decided long ago to end his unhealthy habits and restore vitality and passion to his life. He knows the struggles involved in getting and staying healthy; therefore, he understands the importance of support. *8 Minutes in the Morning* sets you up to win. Jorge is with you each step of the way, but by the end of the 4-week program, the only person you will need is *you*.

8 Minutes in the Morning effectively supports your decision to make health and fitness your top priorities. You will learn how to achieve optimum health and how to attack the process with organization, consistency, and emotion. Time spent exercising is minimized, while your energy is maximized, creating the momentum necessary to propel you toward the body you desire and deserve.

Remember, it is in our moments of decision that our destiny is shaped. I commend and respect you for taking action toward giving yourself the gift of extraordinary health and vitality.

Introduction to a New Life

By Ann-Marie Carpenter, Jorge client and 8 Minute Marvel

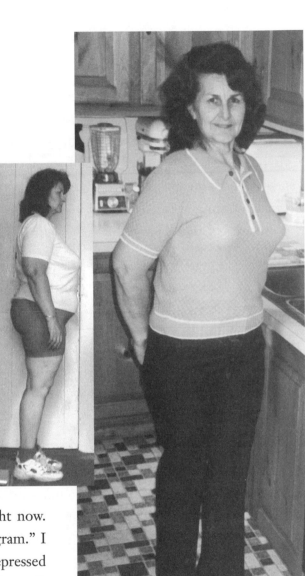

"I lost 2 to 2½ pounds each week—5 pounds every 2 weeks! You can achieve the same results!"

I did nothing for more than 10 years. I felt tired and depressed and weighed 60 pounds more than I should. And it definitely was not extra muscle. Right after I found out that I was a grandmother at age 57, I decided to make sure that I was going to live long enough to not only watch my granddaughter grow up but also have a quality relationship with her. I *had* to lose the weight and get fit, and I had to start immediately.

I know how you may be feeling right now. I had no energy or time to start a "program." I was tired all the time, and I felt more depressed whenever I saw my reflection in the mirror. It had been 15 years since I exercised regularly, followed a healthy diet, or really even thought about weight loss. Back then, I had only 40 pounds to lose. I changed my habits and lost the weight, but within 3 months, I gained it all back, plus 20 pounds. That didn't help my spirits.

Still, I went online to look for a weight-loss plan that I thought I could stick with, and I came across a site that promised me that I could "lose weight and get fit and healthy in only 8 Minutes in the Morning." I figured I would try that. After all, 8 minutes was less time than I spent flipping through channels during TV commercials. The program certainly was a lot cheaper and simpler than all of the potions, pills, and concoctions I'd read about, too. So I ordered Jorge Cruise's program.

Jorge's program made exercising and eating easier. I got fitter, and I lost weight. I was consistently losing—every 2 weeks, I recorded a 5-pound loss! I had lots of energy, and I was feeling great about myself.

Just 5 months later, I had lost 50 pounds. I was down to a size 12 and had not felt deprived for a minute. This program has helped me change my outlook on life. Even after I reached my goal weight, I continued with 8 Minutes in the Morning. Now I am a new me!

I have maintained my weight and my energy level, and Jorge Cruise's program has become a part of my life. The best part about 8 Minutes in the Morning is that anyone can do it. If a grandma at the age of 57 can do it, then anyone can do it! There is nothing magical about my success; *you* can do the same with *8 Minutes in the Morning*. If you make the commitment to take the time for yourself, you can join me in a new life of being fit and healthy, and I guarantee that you will be happier than you have been in a long time.

Thank you, Jorge, for my new life.

Get Ready to Start

Welcome to the ALL-NEW paperback edition of *8 Minutes in the Morning*, the number one weight-loss program for busy people. I want to congratulate you and thank you for selecting me to coach you!

After the hardcover edition hit the *New York Times* bestseller list, I received more and more emails recounting amazing 8 Minutes success stories. I got cmails from people sharing news that they lost two or more pounds each week without fail; raving that following my 8 Minute plan was like discovering the ultimate chocolate cake recipe; and attesting that, like a great recipe, they followed it and got consistent results each time. One woman told me she had become so "delicious" after using 8 Minutes that her husband could not stop nibbling on her. She made me laugh and smile.

How is your life about to change? Why will you get hooked on this program for life? This program is based on the success of more than 3 million of my online "time deprived" clients. I created it based on their feedback and success stories.

So here is my promise to you: **I absolutely guarantee you will lose up to two pounds a week with 8 Minutes if you follow my recipe.** The good news is my plan requires NO trips to the gym, NO counting calories, and NO starvation dieting. Everything you need is in these pages. Plus, I added brand new material on *Emotional Eating* and a few other surprises! So get ready for a new life. I look forward to hearing your success story soon!

Your coach,

JORGE CRUISE

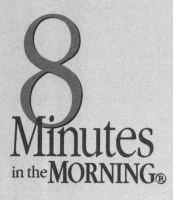
8
Minutes
in the **MORNING**®

PART ONE

Jorge and You

CHAPTER 1

Jorge's Story

The Birth of 8 Minutes in the Morning

There isn't a day that goes by that I don't remember what my life was like before I decided to change my body and make weight loss a priority. I am very grateful when I think of how far I've come. Believe me, it's amazing how great your life can be once you feel good inside and out.

This is why I do what I do. I know that the most valuable instrument you can ever own is a healthy and fit body. No matter what riches you may have, if you are unfit and unhealthy, you have nothing. This is why I have dedicated myself to empowering others with the best and most effective exercise program: my 8 Minutes in the Morning.

You may think that I have always been Mr. Weight Loss, that I have always been addicted to being in great shape, but neither of these things is true. I know what it's like to be embarrassed by extra weight—and worse. I know because *I've been there*. My dad has been there. So have my sister and my grandfather. We were all fat and unhealthy. And now we're not.

The "King" of Poor Health

I grew up in Southern California with a mother from Mexico City and a father from Pennsylvania. Both sides of my family loved rich foods: cheese, milk, cream, anything fried, sausage, and red meat—all served up in huge portions.

Basically, my family had two key beliefs that were wrong. First, they believed that how much you ate equaled how much you were loved. And because my mom and grandma loved me so much, they both fed me a lot. My mom would feed me one meal and then my grandma would almost always offer me another. I showed my love by eating those huge portions. I probably ate enough food for three kids. At home, I consumed enormous quesadillas, bologna sandwiches, and nachos. When we ate out, it was usually at fast-food restaurants, where all my meals were supersized.

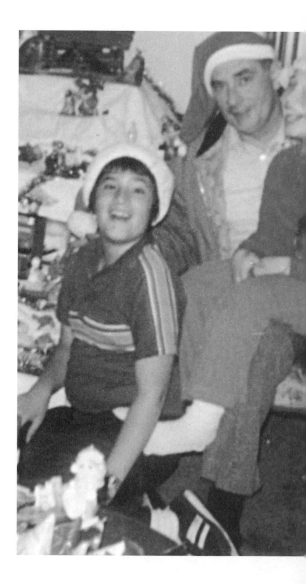

Here I am on the road to an unhealthy life. If I had not changed my eating patterns, I would have easily weighed more than 200 pounds.

If I didn't eat everything on my plate, my mom or grandma would take it very personally. I can't explain why love somehow becomes so intertwined with food. Maybe for my grandmother, it dated back to her childhood years when she was poor and sometimes didn't have enough food. Maybe she wanted to make sure that her grandchildren never had to go through the same kind of childhood.

I got so chubby that my mom used to call me *el rey*, which in Spanish means "the king," and before long, I looked more like King Arthur's table: round.

My family also believed that exercise was hard and time-consuming. My mom and dad were very busy, both working 10-hour days. We *never* exercised. And I don't think anyone in my family ever thought anything was wrong with the way I looked. To my grandmother, the fat on my bones was a sign of health, not a sign of weakness.

Consequently, by the time I was 15, I was a physical disaster. I had low energy, daily headaches, and severe asthma. No one—certainly not my family—ever suspected that my health challenges were caused by my lifestyle.

As I gained weight, I became less active. At school, when it was time to pick teams to play kickball or softball or football, I was always the last kid chosen. I don't think I ever flunked gym class, but I sure didn't do well. I know what it's like to be so unhealthy and unfit that you feel like a reject—a nothing—especially when the kids let you know that they think you're no good. I remember those Presidential Physical Fitness Tests where the gym teacher would make us to do as many situps, pullups, and pushups as we could. I never could do one. Not one.

I went along in this state until I almost died. Yes, you read it right. I had been suffering from a bad stomachache for several weeks. I tried drinking lots of water and herbal teas, but it didn't help. I couldn't eat and quickly started dropping weight. A trip to the emergency room when the pain worsened revealed that a piece of meat had become lodged in my appendix, causing it to burst.

From then on, I tried to change the way I ate, but I didn't know how. The whole concept of healthful eating and exercising was completely foreign to me.

Hitting Too Close to Home

At 18, something happened that made me change my eating and exercise habits for good. My dad was diagnosed with prostate cancer, and the doctors gave him a death sentence. They told him that with no medical intervention, he had 1 year to live. They predicted that if he had his prostate surgically removed and went through a chemotherapy and radiation treatment regimen, he might last 5 to 6 years. My dad knew that surgical removal of his prostate would likely make him incontinent as well as destroy his sex life, so he decided to forgo medical intervention.

That was 1989, and he's still alive and healthy. Instead of undergoing surgery, chemotherapy, and radiation, my dad dramatically changed his lifestyle. He enrolled in

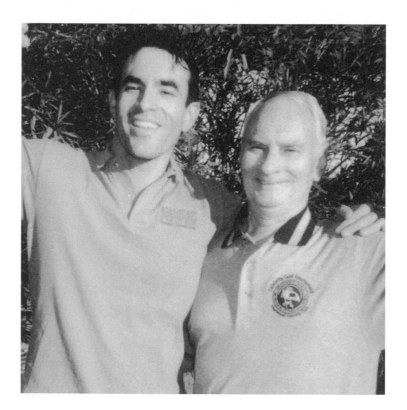

an alternative health center in San Diego where people go to learn about lifestyle changes that promote cleansing, rejuvenating, and healing. I was so shaken up about his cancer that I went with him. I figured that the cancer was probably genetic, and if I didn't take action, I could well be facing the same disease.

Today my dad is 30 pounds lighter and healthier than ever.

At the center, Dad and I learned all about nutrition. We learned which foods contain fiber and which ones don't, about the value of whole grains over processed foods, about fruits and vegetables, about healthful fats, and about herbs such as wheat grass. We discovered that dairy products can cause allergic reactions in some people.

Adopting a New Lifestyle

I stopped eating so much dairy and red meat, switched from processed foods to whole grains and veggies, started drinking more water and eating soy products, and stopped eating supersize hot dogs and hamburgers. One day, I realized that my headaches were gone, and so was my asthma. I was feeling healthy and energetic. I started to exercise, and I enrolled in the University of California, San Diego, to study exercise science and nutrition.

8 Minute Marvel

Marta lost 40 pounds!

BEFORE

Meet Jorge's sister, who joined her brother and father on the path to health.

"I now feel incredible and have attracted the man of my dreams!"

Dad and I weren't the only ones in my family to change our ways. Everyone was turning over a new leaf. Like me, my sister, Marta, had also been an overweight child. She continued to gain weight as she grew older, especially during college. Her weight left her depressed, and her lack of confidence was apparent to everyone who met her. But when she changed her eating habits and started exercising, the weight just fell off. Every time I see her, she's looking more fit and toned.

A Second Chance

In Pennsylvania, my paternal grandparents were dealing with their own problems. They had always followed an unhealthful diet, and when my grandfather retired, they ate even more. They were both significantly overweight, but they didn't think anything of it until my grandmother suffered her first stroke. While she was recovering in the hospital, my grandfather went in for a checkup. The doctor told him to get his affairs in order. At 5 foot 7 inches and 210 pounds, his blood pressure was 180/110, and the doctor assumed that in a short time, he'd be next to have a stroke.

That shook my grandparents up. They knew about my dad's success and decided that adopting his new lifestyle might help them as well. Unfortunately, it was a little too late for my grandmother. They had decided to move to San Diego, but shortly after they arrived, she suffered a second stroke and died.

The new lifestyle showed dramatic results for Grandpa, however. Within months, he dropped more than 50 pounds and lowered his blood pressure to 139/89. He had been given a second chance. At age 95, he feels great, and he and my dad look more like brothers.

A Message of Love

At college, I was busy studying exercise science and swiftly moving from one extreme to the other. I would hit the gym every day, lifting weights that worked the same muscle groups. I knew that exercise was good, but I didn't know that too much could be bad.

I ended up constantly tearing down my muscles and not giving them enough time to recover between sessions. Even though I was eating well and working out, I felt tired all the time. But as my exercise science knowledge grew, I realized that there can be too much of a good thing.

I learned that lesson again a few years later, when my mom—the one person in our family who had lived a fit lifestyle—developed hip problems. In Mexico City, she had been a professional dancer, and in her early sixties, she started feeling more and more hip pain. She was diagnosed

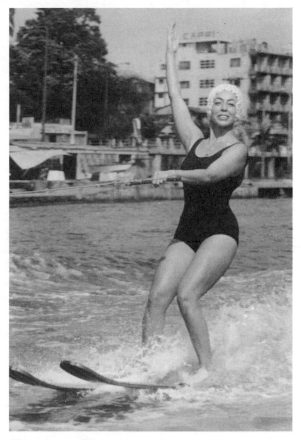

My mom and I were very close, and her passing reinforced my life's mission to empower others.

with osteoarthritis. Essentially, the high-impact dancing she had done most of her life had damaged the cartilage that cushioned her hip joints. Doctors gave her high dosages of painkillers for a year before operating. The painkillers ate away at her kidneys and other body organs. Two years after her hip replacement, my mother died in my arms.

Her death reinforced even more my calling to study exercise science and nutrition. I now know in my heart that my mission in life is to help people get healthy and stay healthy. I want to create a revolution, so I have dedicated my life to empowering others with the best and most effective weight-loss information. This is why I became certified as a fitness trainer by the Cooper Institute for Aerobics Research, the American College of Sports Medicine (ACSM), and the American Council on Exercise (ACE).

About the Program

After getting the know-how, I created www.jorgecruise.com, my weight-loss Web site. Within weeks of launching it, I was helping thousands make the same lifestyle changes that had worked for me and for my family. My site became so successful that Oprah Winfrey invited me to appear on her show. She surprised me by inviting two people to appear on the show who had transformed their lives with the help of the information on my site.

After that show, my online business and career took off. Soon, millions visited the site regularly, trying the techniques I suggested and giving me feedback about what worked for them and what didn't. People told me that with their work and families, they just didn't have time for long trips to the gym, hour-long aerobics sessions, or complicated eating plans. They wanted simplicity.

How It Works

Follow my 8 Minutes in the Morning program and you will see amazing weight-loss results in just 28 days. But it doesn't stop there. I will also give you the tools you need to stay lean for the rest of your life. You will be working on three things every day:

Your emotional fitness. Before your 8 Minutes in the Morning routine, I will help you build your own inner motivation with my daily Wake-Up Talk. It will give you the Emotional Advantage you need to move beyond self-sabotaging thinking and motivate yourself to love your new fit lifestyle.

Your physical fitness. My proven "two superquick moves" are the center of the program. They take only 8 minutes a day, but the results are tremendous. Each day, I will give you two new strength-training moves specifically designed to help you speed up your metabolism, get firm, and burn fat as efficiently as possible. (See illustration on page 11.)

Your eating habits. My Eat Fat to Get Fit nutrition program is simple to follow and will never leave you feeling deprived. You won't have to count calories or cut out your favorite foods.

Finally, 8 Minutes in the Morning connects you to a community of your peers. I invite you to visit my Web site at www.jorgecruise.com to get more advice from me and to chat with the millions of others who, like you, are well on their way to achieving new health and happiness.

I made a deal with some of these clients. I would train them personally as long as they allowed me to experiment on them. They would

have to try exercises, eating plans, and a motivational program that I would give them. In exchange, they had to let me know what worked and what did not. The result was 8 Minutes in the Morning.

My Web site also started to address the needs of busy people. I wrote articles and did Webcasts about time-efficient exercise programs and then sought feedback from my clients. Together, we shaped the program into an overwhelming success.

Will 8 Minutes in the Morning do the same for you? Absolutely. You will see guaranteed rapid weight loss when you follow my program. It does not take a lot of time to get lean as long as you consistently use the most effective exercises. 8 Minutes in the Morning is all you need.

The Truth About Fat

Muscle loss begins with inactivity as shown in the cross-sections of thighs (by magnetic imaging). As inactive muscle breaks down, fat builds up. Only strength training can restore youthful fat-burning muscle tissue.

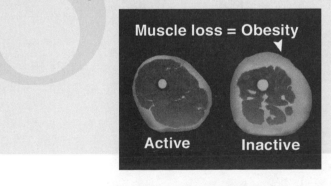

Muscle loss = Obesity

Active   Inactive

Why You Are Fat

We Have All Been Misled

Since the early 1980s, when the term *aerobics* came into vogue, hundreds of exercise programs have been launched to help people get lean. Perhaps you've tried step aerobics, slide aerobics, kickbox aerobics, or even just walking, jogging, or running.

Despite all the publicity these different aerobics programs have received over the years, Americans are still fat—and they're getting fatter at an alarming rate. According to *Newsweek*, in 1991, only four states had obesity rates of more than 14 percent of their populations. By 1998, 37 of 50 states had surpassed that threshold. Currently, more than 80 percent of the total U.S. population is overweight. And nearly one-quarter are clinically obese.

And it's not just here in America. According to the Worldwatch Institute, the figure is 54 per-

The Consequences of Obesity

Obesity increases the risk for the following:

- Premature death
- High blood pressure
- Diabetes and insulin resistance
- Gallbladder disease
- Kidney disease
- Liver disease
- Heart disease
- Many types of cancer

- Arthritis
- Orthopedic disorders
- Fatal respiratory disease
- Stroke
- Gout
- Asthma
- Back pain
- Shortness of breath
- Sleep apnea and snoring

- Reproductive disorders (menstrual problems, female infertility, miscarriage, gestational diabetes)
- Unhealthy cholesterol levels
- Impaired immune function
- Depression
- Chronic pain
- Impaired mobility

cent in Russia; in the United Kingdom, 51 percent; and in Germany, 50 percent. What is even sadder is that juvenile obesity is also rising rapidly. In the United States, the incidence of obesity among children has more than doubled over the last 30 years.

According to former Surgeon General C. Everett Koop and the Center for Disease Control and Prevention (CDC), more than 300,000 Americans die each year from obesity-related illnesses—second only to 400,000 for tobacco. This means each day, over 800 Americans die from problems related to obesity.

That is the equivalent of 6 airliners with 133 people on board fatally crashing daily. This means that just within this next hour, 34 Americans will die. Think about it . . . about every 5 minutes, three people die due to problems related to obesity. And according to Jeffrey D. Koplan, M.D., director of the CDC, "This dramatic new evidence signals the unfolding of an epidemic in the United States." Unbelievably, Americans have the lowest life expectancy of all industrialized nations.

The average woman gains 9 pounds between her 30th and 39th birthdays; the average man gains 4. It is these types of extra pounds that put you at an increased risk for disease. (See "The Consequences of Obesity.") It is estimated by the World Health Organization that up to one-third of cancers of the colon, breast, prostate, kidney, and digestive tract are due to obesity and lack of exercise. The bottom line is that the fatter you are, the higher your chance of dying prematurely.

Why Aerobics Is Not the Most Effective

Although aerobic exercise is essential for strengthening your heart and lungs (the cardiovascular system), it is not the most effective way to get lean. You burn roughly 100 calories for every mile that you walk or run. To lose 1 pound, you would have to walk or run 35 miles.

And aerobic exercise is not so practical if you are overweight. It can be too uncomfortable. Even walking can be difficult because your joints may start to ache, and you can become winded very quickly. Before coming to me, almost all of my clients had given up exercising because the aerobic approach was too difficult for them. Plus, if you focus on aerobics, your body shape will stay the same, even if you burn enough body fat. If you are currently shaped like a pear, you will look like a smaller pear. You'll lose weight first where you don't want to—your breasts—and last where you do want to—your thighs. Your body will still feel flabby and, worse, your skin will probably sag.

But the exercises in my 8 Minutes in the Morning program will help you burn fat and improve your body shape. You will tone your shoulders so that your waist looks narrower. Your arms will be smaller as well as firmer. Your abdominal muscles will be not only leaner but stronger, and they'll provide better support for your torso.

I'm not saying that you shouldn't do *any* aerobic exercise. Beyond my 8 Minutes, I recommend that you incorporate some aerobics into your lifestyle because you need to keep your heart and lungs strong. Plus, it reduces stress. For tips on beginning the most convenient type of aerobic exercise, see the chapter on powerwalking on page 199.

Why Starvation Dieting Doesn't Work

You have been told that dieting is the key to weight loss, that weight loss is simple—just don't eat. And research shows that you can fairly easily lose unwanted weight by starving yourself. The problem is that up to 50 percent of that weight comes from muscle tissue loss, not from fat loss. This sets you up for disaster.

Here's what happens. When you don't eat enough, your thyroid gland (located in your neck) tries to protect you from starvation. It secretes less thyroxine, a hormone that helps regulate your metabolism. The less thyroxine you have, the slower your metabolism and the fewer calories you burn. If you continue this stringent diet for a long period of time, your body will eventually start to consume itself. You may think that this is wonderful because, after all, you *do* want to slim down. But half of that weight loss will have come from lean muscle tissue.

Your muscle tissue is your body's metabolic furnace. Every pound of muscle burns roughly 50 calories a day. Every pound of muscle you lose on a diet means that your metabolism slows by 50 calories a day. As your metabolism slows down, you'll have to eat less and less food to compensate. Eventually, weight loss becomes extremely difficult and you hit that all-too-familiar plateau. Few people can continue to eat so few calories for any length of time. As soon as you start eating normally again, your body will regain the weight you just lost. And because nearly all of that regained weight goes straight to your fat cells, your metabolism will stay just as sluggish. This is why many people who lose weight end up gaining back more than they originally lost.

For many people, muscle is already in perilously short supply. What you don't use, you lose. And a convenience-driven lifestyle of escalators, remote controls, and drive-thru coffee shops takes a huge toll on your muscle mass over time. As you lose muscle, your metabolism grows more sluggish. This is why people tend to grow fatter as they age. Even if you don't gain weight, you may still get fatter because heavier, more compact muscle tissue is replaced by lighter, more expansive fat tissue. You weigh the same when you get on the scale, but your pants no longer fit.

Fortunately, there is a better way. If starving yourself and huffing and puffing through hours of aerobics didn't give you the belly, butt, and thighs—or the health benefits—of your dreams, then it's time to try the most efficient and quickest way to get lean: my special combination of superquick strength-training moves and the Eat Fat to Get Fit eating system.

CHAPTER 3

The Emotional Advantage

Your Firm Foundation

To lose weight with 8 Minutes in the Morning, you must first get what I call an Emotional Advantage. In my work with millions of clients online, I've learned that emotional and physical health go hand in hand. Most people can't lose weight and keep it off until they also lose their negative emotions. Once they get fit emotionally, it's like magic. Everything else becomes just a walk in the park.

So no matter what genetic deck of cards you have been dealt, an Emotional Advantage will help to ensure you have a *successful and fun weight-loss journey*. With it, you will not only lose weight and build strength but also you will feel your confidence soar.

How can I guarantee that you will really lose the weight this time, and keep it off? Well, millions of my online clients have been exactly where you are, and now they are fit and firm.

Danny Chacon did it. So did Sam Raymond, Eva Rushing, Scott Vuola, Stephanie Donald, George Wingerd, and many, many more.

Full, but Not Fulfilled

I'd like to tell you a story about Amber Dunlap, a client who was one of my first Emotional Advantage test cases. She started dieting when she was in high school, gaining and losing the same 10 to 15 pounds in an effort to become thin enough to be a model. "I was miserable. I was constantly depressed and struggling to keep the pounds off," she told me.

As the years went by, her depression magnified and her weight increased. "I decided that if I were going to get big, I might as well eat all of the foods that I had denied myself for so long." And she did.

8 Minute Marvel
Amber lost 21 pounds!

BEFORE

"It was the easiest weight I ever lost. I love that it only takes me 8 minutes in the morning to do my routine."

Amber was also featured on the cover of *Woman's World* magazine. See her weight-loss success at jorgecruise.com

"Then one day, I caught a glimpse of myself in a glass door. I saw more than an out-of-shape woman. I saw an empty soul. I felt so unfulfilled, and I had no idea how to change it."

After spending 4 weeks building her Emotional Advantage, she told me, "Emotionally, I feel so in control. This program helped me change my old self-sabotaging habits to ones that support my growth. The mental exercises have helped me look into my heart and soul to find what I need in this life. I have faith in myself and my ability to change what I can for my success."

Getting Fit from the Inside Out

Think of all the exercise and weight-loss programs that you have started—and then stopped. At the beginning, you felt so confident, so excited, so sure that this time you were going to see results. This time you were *not* going to fall off the weight-loss wagon.

How long did that feeling last? Two weeks? Three weeks? Or just 2 days? For any exercise or weight-loss program to work, you must stay with it. I'm going to teach you how to make the positive feelings last much longer—for the rest of your life. You will see dramatic weight loss in just 4 weeks, and you will get hooked on doing the 8 Minutes in the Morning program. I guarantee that your motivational drive will grow stronger every day with a simple system to keep you focused so that you stay *consistently* inspired to take action.

IDENTIFY! DISCOVER! TRANSFORM!

You will become more fit on the outside by firming up and losing fat, but you'll also become fit on the inside. And when you get fit from the inside out, you'll tap storehouses of motivation and confidence that you didn't know you had.

Think about it. If you perceive exercise as a chore, odds are that you won't exercise consistently. If you think of eating well as punishment, you probably won't eat well consistently. How you *feel* controls your behavior and directly affects your physical fitness. When something makes you feel extraordinary, you do it effortlessly. If you feel unfocused, unmotivated, and tired, you don't.

Will you snack on an apple or a piece of cheesecake? Will you wake up early to exercise or sleep in? Go for a vigorous walk or drop in front of the TV after work? The key to automatically choosing the healthier option is knowing how to manage your emotions. That's where the Emotional Advantage comes in.

Your Wake-Up Talk

Each day, before you start your 8 Minutes in the Morning strength-training moves, you'll spend a few minutes getting focused and emotionally inspired with a Wake-Up Talk. These will infuse your strength training with the Emotional Advantage and help you feel consistently motivated to take action. Through these talks, you will:

• Identify your weight-loss goals—IDENTIFY!
• Discover new incentives for shedding those pounds—DISCOVER!
• Transform yourself from a negative thinker into a positive thinker—TRANSFORM!

- Create a secret energy source by changing the way you breathe
- Use the power of visualization to change your actions
- Free up time that you didn't know you had
- Boost your mood in just 1 second
- Unveil your self-confidence

These short talks will change your outlook on life. Until now, you've been thinking like a fat person. Your Wake-Up Talks will teach you how to think like a thin person. These talks take just a few moments each day to do, but by the end of the initial month-long program, you'll feel happy, confident, driven, committed, and focused. The Emotional Advantage will help you not only stick with the 8 Minutes in the Morning program but it will actually help you look forward to it!

The Write Stuff

In addition to your morning Wake-Up Talk, you'll find Today's Journal—another daily feature of the 8 Minutes in the Morning program. Use this space to record your progress, your breakthroughs, and what you are grateful for in your life. This book is meant to be interactive and cannot be finalized without your input. Writing your goals and thoughts will personalize your program. It's a simple yet effective process. One of the most powerful ways you learn is from yourself, and keeping a journal will teach you more about you. So keep a pen handy and add your notes to each day's journal. When you add the information that is uniquely yours, this book automatically becomes the most important book in your library.

> Today's Journal
> Today was great. I got up early enough to do the program and actually eat breakfast at home instead of at work. I want to try to do this more often...it starts my day much more calmly. Jan asked me to run a few errands with her at lunch, so I suggested we walk instead of drive. We got our aerobic activity in at the same time! I did eat chocolate today, but only 2 of those miniature-size bars, so I feel good about that. All in all, it was a great day... if I keep it up, I'll be in that new shorts outfit at next weekend's get-together. I'm looking forward to what my relatives and friends will think of the new me!

When I started using journaling as part of my program, there was an overwhelming response from my clients. It became a permanent positive feature of 8 Minutes in the

Morning. Perhaps Oprah Winfrey said it best: "Keeping a journal will absolutely change your life in ways you've never imagined."

Use your journal to write about:

- How you feel
- Your energy level
- What you did great today, such as a positive thought you had or a positive action ("I had some candy-coated chocolates today and stopped at just three!")
- The foods you ate or any new recipes you tried
- How you are progressing in the program (include the details)
- The positive benefits of your continuing weight loss ("Bob told me I looked great today.")

Use this journal as a log of your personal journey. Whether you write a paragraph or fill up a page, get in the habit of listening to your inner thoughts and writing about how you feel. After the 4-week program, I'm going to ask you to read through your journal entries so that you can see how far you've come.

Getting Started

To jump-start the building of your inner emotional strength, do the following three simple things right now.

Take Your "Before" Photo

Most people tell me that they hate having their "before" photos taken. What they mean is that they hate having *any* photos of themselves taken. Yet my clients often e-mail me and thank me for having encouraged them to do it. Having that photo taken is such a basic action, yet it signals a change deep inside you. As soon as that photo is developed, it becomes the "before" photo, starting you on your journey to your "after" photo.

It's such a simple distinction, but such a strong symbol. You would not believe how many of my clients tell me how their attitudes about weight loss changed almost instantly just because they took that "before" picture. It's a symbol of your commitment. It's a symbol of your new beginning.

Tips from the Photo Pros

It is in your best interest to take a great "before" photo. The better the quality of the photo, the more accurately you'll be able to assess your progress.

1. Have your photo fill the frame as much as possible without cutting off body parts.
2. Use a quality camera and film.
3. Use a background that is medium to light in color.
4. Take the picture in good light, either in the early morning or late evening.
5. Keep the camera angle the same on your "before" and "after" photos.
6. Use the same pose as you will for your "after" photo.
7. Keep your original photo and negatives in a safe location.

Your photo is a powerful reminder of your progress, and that's motivating! Clients say that on their worst days, they would look at their "before" photos and feel instantly inspired.

Finally, that photo will hold you accountable to the program. Your "before" photo is one of the most important tools you will ever use. It will remind you of your amazing progress for years to come. You will remain grateful and inspired for life. Look at it periodically and tell yourself, "That's the old me." Your "new me" is finally emerging!

Decide What You Want

Clarity is power. You need to have focus to achieve your goals, according to author Tony Robbins, my friend and mentor. He taught me that to get what you want in life, you must first know what you *specifically* want. Too often, he says, if you ask someone what she wants, you'll hear instead about what she doesn't want.

To illustrate his point, he shared this story. Tony was invited to learn how to drive a race car. He was surprised to learn that most injuries come from not successfully coming out of spins. His instructor told him that the key to coming out of a spin is to focus on

Tracking Your Success

Before you go any further, take the time to assess where you are now so you can compare it with where you'll be. This is another really good thing to do that all my clients love. You will, too.

Tape your "before" photo here. (Double-sided tape works best.)

Today's date: _____

Body Measurements

Right arm:_____ Left arm:_____

Bust/Chest:_____ Neck:_____

Waist:_____ Hips:_____

Right thigh:_____ Left thigh:_____

Weight:_____

Tape your "after" photo here.

Today's date: _____

Body Measurements

Right arm:_____ Left arm:_____

Bust/Chest:_____ Neck:_____

Waist:_____ Hips:_____

Right thigh:_____ Left thigh:_____

Weight:_____

where you want to go. Instead, most people focus on what they fear—the wall—and so that's where they go.

Even though Tony had been told this, the first time he went into a spin, his eyes went right to the wall. His instructor had to grab his head and move it to where the car needed to go. Sure enough, as he focused in that direction, he couldn't help but turn the steering wheel accordingly.

Weight loss is a lot like driving that race car. In order to get results, you must focus on where you want to go. Saying what you don't want—"I don't want to be fat"—is not going to get you there. That's like looking at the wall. To get what you want, you must focus on what you want. Yet saying "I want to lose weight" is not as effective as saying, "I want to lose 10 pounds this month." The second gives you clarity and focus. It also gives you a deadline.

But don't choose your goal randomly. It must be realistic. To estimate your ideal weight, look at "Finding Your Ideal Weight." Once you know your goal weight and the approximate date you will achieve it, keep yourself motivated by doing the following.

Weigh yourself every week. Don't be afraid to get on the scale. It is important for you to track your weight-loss progress. Weigh in on *Sundays*, ideally first thing in the morning before you eat. Your weight may fluctuate due to water retention and the amount of food in your stomach, so don't sweat it if every once in a while it seems as though you haven't made much progress.

To see your true progress, use the "Success Chart" on page 26. Use it to plot your weight loss each week. Once you connect the dots, you'll see that, overall, your weight is dropping.

Use a tape measure. It's helpful for you to track the inches you are losing. This will keep you motivated and on track. Remember that muscle is more compact than fat, and you will be increasing your lean muscle tissue as you burn away fat. You will be replacing fat with muscle, so you will see a significant difference in inches even if you don't see a dramatic loss in pounds. Your clothes will feel looser as you become fitter. Measure just

Finding Your Ideal Weight

Find your age and height on the chart. You know yourself better than anyone else does, so select a number that is realistic for you. Subtract that number from your current weight. That's your weight-loss goal. Write the number on this line:

_____

 Figure out a target date for achieving your weight-loss goal. On the 8 Minutes in the Morning program, you can expect to lose fat at a sensible and safe rate of 1½ to 2 pounds a week, which is what doctors recommend. Some people lose 3 to 4 pounds in a week. So to lose 55 pounds of fat, it will take you 20 to 25 weeks. That means sticking to the program for only 5 to 6 months. The great news is that you will start to see results in just 28 days.

 Divide the amount of weight you want to lose by 2 (the average number of pounds most people lose each week). The result is the number of weeks it should take you to reach your goal weight. Write this number and the date by which you will achieve this new weight on the line below. (Get your calendar out if you need to and find the date.)

_____ pounds by _____ [date]

Height (ft/in.)	Weight (lb) 19-34 yr	35+ yr	Height (ft/in.)	Weight (lb) 19-34 yr	35+ yr
5'0"	97–128	108–38	5'8"	125–64	138–78
5'1"	101–32	111–43	5'9"	129–69	142–83
5'2"	104–37	115–48	5'10"	132–74	146–88
5'3"	107–41	119–52	5'11"	136–79	151–94
5'4"	111–46	122–57	6'0"	140–84	155–99
5'5"	114–50	126–62	6'1"	144–89	159–205
5'6"	118–55	130–67	6'2"	148–95	164–210
5'7"	121–60	134–72	6'3"	152–200	168–216

SOURCE: U.S. Department of Health and Human Services, *Dietary Guideline for Americans*

Success Chart

Starting at zero, chart your weight loss on the graph. The horizontal line lists weeks and the vertical line keeps a running total of pounds lost or gained.

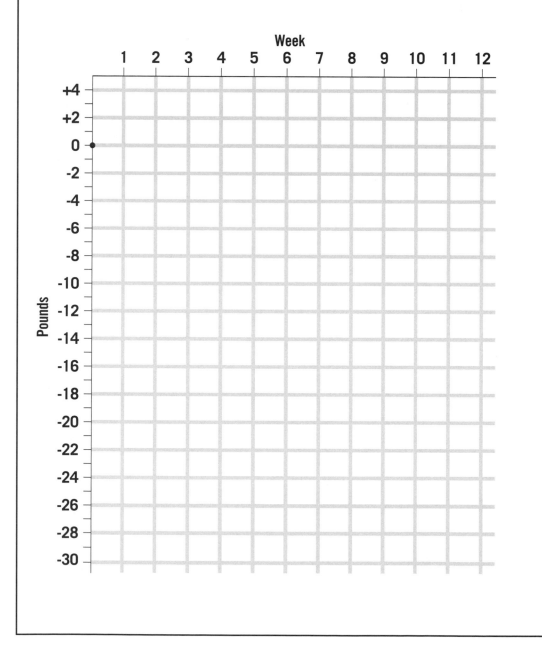

below your belly button and any other areas you want to monitor, such as your thighs, arms, or neck.

Look at yourself in a full-length mirror. Don't think of the mirror as your enemy. Use it to see your fat changing to muscle, noticing the definition you are gaining in your muscles. The longer you stick with the program, the better you'll look.

Commit Yourself to Success

Too many people commit themselves only half-heartedly to losing weight. They tell themselves, "Well, if this works out, great, but if not, it's no big deal." And they don't tell anyone that they are dieting because that way, if they fail, no one has to know about it.

The problem with that approach is that without commitment and support, you'll have a tough time sticking to a program. People may unknowingly sabotage your efforts by bringing you gifts of food. Or your spouse may expect you to stay up late at night with him, making it difficult for you to get up early for your exercises. And when things are rough, you won't have anyone there to tell you, "You can't stop now."

That's why I want you to fill out "My Success Contract" on page 28 right now. It may feel

Frequently Asked Questions

How can I be sure that I'll stick with 8 Minutes in the Morning?

Send me a copy of the contract that you filled out and signed on page 28. I would be honored to acknowledge your commitment to a healthier and happier lifestyle, and I will do what I can to hold you to it. E-mail your Success Contract to contract@jorgecruise.com or find my mailing address at www.jorgecruise.com/mail.

Please be sure to include your name, address, phone number, and e-mail address because I might even call you on your target date to see how you did. Knowing that I could call you should help you stay on track!

My Success Contract

8 Minutes® in the MORNING

8 Minutes® in the MORNING

Filling out this contract is one of the important first steps in the 8 Minutes in the Morning program. Make three copies and give them to trusted friends who will support and motivate you in your journey to success.

Name: _____

Today's date: _____

I am going to lose this many pounds: _____

By this date: _____

_____
Signature

8 Minutes® in the MORNING

8 Minutes® in the MORNING

a little odd, but it's a powerful reminder of your decision and will hold you accountable to the program.

Once you fill out the contract, make three photocopies. I strongly recommend that you give the copies to people you feel you can trust, and share your plans with them. Explain to them how you intend to lose the weight, and tell them how they can help. Following are a couple of tips for talking to friends and family about your goal.

Be open. Often, just sitting your spouse and kids down for a heart-to-heart talk is all you need. Tell them how they can help you, and how they are not helping you now. Explain how their actions—eating potato chips in front of you, putting you down because of your weight—make you feel. Talk about how your current weight makes you feel, and how being your goal weight will make you feel so much better. Tell your family specific things they can do to make your journey easier. Maybe they can eat their chips in another room, or maybe they can do the program with you.

Compromise. Spouses and children sometimes hinder weight-loss efforts simply because it's inconvenient for them. Ask them to help you come up with a compromise. Remember that you are in charge. You have the power to make your decisions. No one but you can make you eat something you don't want to eat. No one but you can force you to skip your 8 Minutes in the Morning.

Also make sure to discover my new secrets on Eliminating Emotional Eating. (See page 235).

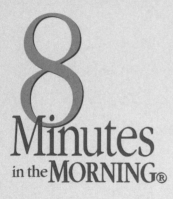

PART TWO

How It Works

CHAPTER 4

Two Superquick Moves and You're Done!

Getting Lean Fast

It's no wonder that people think exercising is too hard and takes too much time. During various attempts to lose weight and firm up, they have forced themselves to sweat it out for a half-hour or more, and worst of all, saw few results. It does *not* take a lot of time to get lean if you consistently use the most effective exercises. And just a couple of the right efficient fat-burning moves will give you unbelievable results. This is the core of my 8 Minutes in the Morning program.

The most effective exercise program for losing weight is a morning strength-training session. This is absolutely critical for you to know! Your true problem is not excess fat; that's just the symptom. The underlying problem is a lack of lean muscle tissue. Why? The single most important factor that determines how much fat you burn throughout the

Your "8 Minutes" Edge

Strength training is the smart way to lose weight because it's also good for your overall health. New research shows that strength training:

• Increases bone density, helping to prevent osteoporosis

• Improves your balance, preventing falls and injuries

• Lowers your blood pressure, cholesterol levels, and risk of stroke, diabetes, cancer, and arthritis

• Boosts your metabolism to burn fat 24 hours a day

• Raises energy levels for a more active lifestyle

• Promotes a better mood and better sleep patterns with the release of endorphins

• Brings an end to yo-yo weight loss and gain

day is the amount of lean muscle tissue in your body. The more lean muscle tissue you have, the more efficiently your body burns fat. (See chapter 5, starting on page 40, to understand the fat-burning power of the morning.)

Rev Up Your Fat Burner

Imagine that you are a Volkswagen Beetle but your mechanic has upgraded your engine to a more powerful one from a Porsche. Would this stronger engine consume more fuel? Yes. The same is true when you strength train. You create more muscle (a stronger engine) and burn more fat (your fuel).

In addition to creating stronger muscles, strength training also creates a stronger metabolism. That's because lean muscle tissue is very "active," and requires more calories to survive. Lean muscle tissue is a "calorie eater" and will help you get and keep a lean body. The more lean muscle tissue you have, the more body fat you will burn!

Imagine you added 5 pounds of lean muscle tissue over the next few months. (Pound for pound, muscle takes up a lot less space than fat.) You would then be burning an additional 250 calories a day without changing your diet. That means that you would be burning over

25 pounds of fat each year you maintain the muscle. And remember that on my program, you will be building up lean muscle tissue and following my Eat Fat to Get Fit nutritional program. When you put these two components together, you will see guaranteed results—an average of a 2-pound weight loss each week. Normally, when you lose weight, you lose 75 percent of it as fat and 25 percent of it as muscle. But when you do strength training, you lose nearly all fat and no muscle. Lean tissue derives 75 to 95 percent of its energy from body fat, so for every new pound of muscle you build, you incinerate about 50 additional calories per day. The more lean tissue you have, the more body fat you will shed—even at night, while you sleep. So instead of burning just 60 calories of fat per hour while sitting in a chair at work, you now burn 120 calories of fat per hour doing the same thing.

Feel Younger and Stronger

Besides looking better, you're going to feel better, too. You'll feel younger because strength training turns back the aging clock. According to a study of postmenopausal women, the body becomes 15 to 20 years more youthful after just 1 year of strength training. Strength training also encourages you to exercise more throughout the day.

And once your muscles become stronger—usually by week 2 or 3—you will find yourself suddenly doing things you never thought possible. You'll opt to take a walk in the evening instead of sitting in front of the television, you'll want to take the stairs at work, and you'll get up from behind that desk to take quick walking breaks throughout

Frequently Asked Questions

Will the strength-training exercises in your 8 Minutes in the Morning program make me look like a weight lifter?

Ladies, don't worry about bulking up. Women don't produce as much of the growth-producing hormone testosterone as men do—men produce up to 30 times more. Female bodybuilders follow a very different training program and achieve "he-man" looks only with steroid use. I promise that your muscles will become firmer, sexier, and shapelier—not bulkier.

your workday. You'll ignore escalators, elevators, and moving walkways in favor of your own two feet. All of this will accelerate your results.

And remember what I said about aerobic exercise being too challenging when you're overweight? That's not true for strength training. There will be no uncomfortable huffing and puffing with my program. Apart from a few sets of dumbbells, you will need no special clothing or equipment, either. Even if you have never succeeded in losing 1 pound with aerobics or other exercise programs, I guarantee that you'll do great with 8 Minutes in the Morning—and that 8 Minutes in the Morning will make you feel great!

Frequently Asked Questions

While I have the weights in my hands, can I add some repetitions to increase the effects of my 8 Minutes in the Morning workouts?

The strength-training exercises included in the 8 Minutes in the Morning program are designed to work in sync with the nutritional intake values that are indicated with the Eating Card System (see page 70). A better fitness move for you is to challenge your body with aerobic activities, starting with my powerwalking program on page 199.

How Strength Training Works

Once you start my 28-day program, you'll work two different groups of muscles each day. Sunday is your day off.

Monday: Chest and back

Tuesday: Shoulders and abdominals

Wednesday: Triceps and biceps (arms)

Thursday: Hamstrings and quadriceps (legs)

Friday: Calves and butt

Saturday: Inner and outer thighs

Each day of the program brings you two new exercises. And this is one of the most unique aspects of the 8 Minutes in the Morning program. The way I've combined these exercises allows you to consistently challenge your muscles in new ways. Each day, you'll break down muscle tissue, which is a good thing. It's how your body grows. After your workout, your body goes to work to repair that lean tissue, making you stronger. The next time you lift the same weight, it won't feel so heavy.

This muscle-repair stage is called the afterburn. Your metabolism will stay revved up for hours after your 8 Minutes in the Morning—7 to 12 percent higher for 15 or more hours, which amounts to 600-plus incinerated calories. After you do aerobic exercise, your metabolism returns to normal within an hour, burning only 15 to 50 additional calories.

Choose Your Weights

To do your 8 Minutes in the Morning exercises, all you'll need are some dumbbells, a chair, and a towel or mat.

I strongly recommend that you purchase three pairs of dumbbells: a light pair, a medium pair, and a heavy pair. This will ensure that you work both your smaller and larger muscles effectively. To figure out which weights to buy, take the biceps curl test.

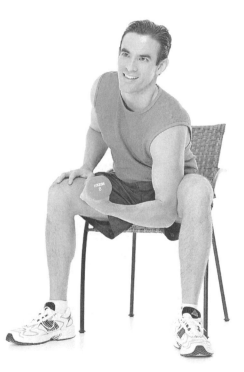

1. Select a weight that you think you can curl 12 times without stopping.
2. With a dumbbell in each hand, repeatedly curl the weight.
3. If you can curl more than 12 times, the weight is too light. If you can't reach 12 repetitions, the weight is too heavy. If you can do 12 repetitions but not 13, you've found the right middle-range weight.

What Makes 8 Minutes of Strength Training So Smart?

The type of strength training in my program is perfect for busy people. Here are just a few of the unique reasons why 8 Minutes in the Morning is the most effective way to lose weight.

• My program encourages you to strength train in the morning. When you strength train in the morning, as opposed to later in the day, you will immediately elevate your metabolism for the whole day. After your 8 Minutes in the Morning session, your body will be working hard to start building your lean tissue, and that will seriously boost your metabolism. And that's only one of many benefits of morning exercise.

• Other strength-training programs have you spend 40 minutes or more in the gym, but my program contains a special series of moves that take only 8 minutes a day. I specifically designed and tested this workout based on the feedback of millions of my online clients. They told me that they didn't have time for the trip to the gym and that they wanted to work out at home without buying fancy equipment.

• My proven moves are the most efficient combination of strength-training moves around. I tested them on my online clients. They work. By consistently challenging different muscle groups every day, you'll give your metabolism the biggest boost possible.

• I have combined my strength-training moves with two other bonus components that will further maximize your weight loss. I call the first one the Emotional Advantage. It's the motivational component of 8 Minutes in the Morning, and it will keep you on track. The second is my breakthrough eating program called Eat Fat to Get Fit. For guaranteed success on your 8 Minutes in the Morning program, you must use all three aspects of the program at the same time.

4. To select your lighter weights, subtract 2 to 3 pounds from your middle-range weight. For example, if you selected 8 pounds as your mid-range dumbbell, you would most likely select a 5- or 6-pound dumbbell as your lighter one.

5. To select your heavier dumbbell, add 2 to 3 pounds to your mid-range dumbbell. If your mid-range weight were 8 pounds, you should most likely select a 10-pound dumbbell. (It is rare to find 11-pound dumbbells.)

You can find suitable dumbbells in most sporting-goods stores. Or try my favorite dumbbell system at www.powerblock.com. It provides several weight options with a single pair of dumbbells. You'll love it!

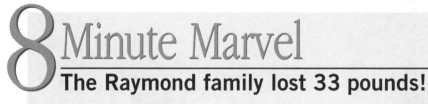

8 Minute Marvel

The Raymond family lost 33 pounds!

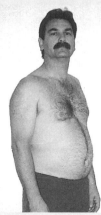

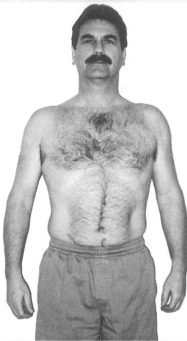

SAM BEFORE

"After we found Jorge's program, we decided to make it a family project. This is something that we can all benefit from and support each other in. We get up and do the exercises together, which takes less than 15 minutes a day! We're getting active as a family, which has enriched our lives and brought us closer. So far, Sam has lost 16 pounds, I have lost 10, and Nicolas has lost 7. We have more strength and energy, and even sleep better."

—Carrie Raymond

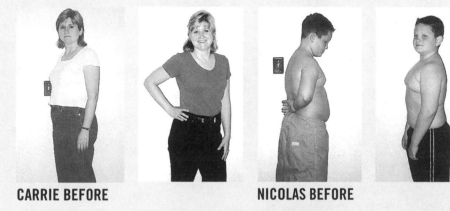

CARRIE BEFORE

NICOLAS BEFORE

CHAPTER 5

Roll Out of Bed to a New You

Why Move in the Morning?

When I suggest to people that they get up 8 minutes earlier in the morning to exercise, I sometimes get: "Oh, I'm not a morning person. That will never work for me. As soon as the alarm goes off, I'll hit the snooze button." If you keep thinking that way, that's what you'll do.

I truly believe that there's no such thing as not being a morning person; that's all in your head. I used to stay up late at night because I thought of myself as a night owl. Our thoughts are powerful, and they control our actions. I would read, watch television, listen to music, and talk to friends on the phone. So when I first started exercising in the morning, I had a really tough time doing it consistently. It's hard to get out of bed in the morning when you just crawled *into* bed a few hours before.

But I was motivated to turn things around. I only had to remind myself of Dad's bout with prostate cancer, my grandmother's death from a stroke, and Grandpa's scare with high blood pressure to motivate myself to get a proper night's sleep. And when I exercised in the morning, I felt wonderful for the rest of the day. Now I don't stay up later than 10:00 P.M., and I'm out of bed by 6 in the morning.

Rise and Shine

Consider the case of Lisa Kasirye, one of my online clients. She works 9:30 A.M. to 6:00 P.M. After work, she cooks, cleans, and sometimes at-

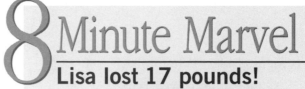

8 Minute Marvel
Lisa lost 17 pounds!

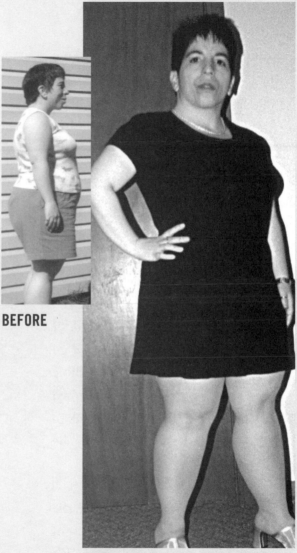

BEFORE

"Once I got started, I just wanted to do more. It's great to want to walk up the stairs or to the corner store rather than drive."

tends night classes. When I first met Lisa, she didn't even start thinking about getting ready for bed until after 10:00 P.M. At the beginning of her program, she told me that she slept exhaustedly until 8:30 every morning. She slept away most of her weekends. She couldn't imagine a good reason for getting up any earlier.

But then Lisa committed to 8 Minutes in the Morning. At first, she got up only 15 minutes earlier than usual. After only a couple of weeks on the program, she had lost weight and her energy level had skyrocketed. "I have the energy to work out *and* go walking. I enjoy it! This incredible energy is something I never dreamed of. I'm so revitalized that I want to participate in life to the fullest," she told me.

After 9 weeks on the program, she had lost 17 pounds. "Once I got started, I just wanted to do more. It's great to want to walk up the stairs or walk to the corner store rather than drive," she said.

8 Minute Marvel
Howard lost 91 pounds!

"For me, the program creates wonderful results without struggle. I indulge in chocolate on occasion—my fat-burning metabolism easily burns the extra calories."

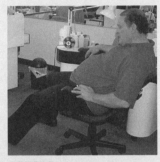

BEFORE

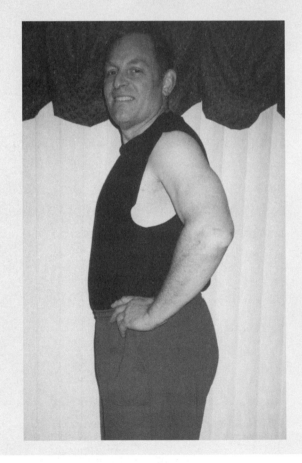

If you think Lisa is an exception, think again. My program affected Howard Joseph the same way.

Howard worked 12- to 14-hour shifts as a professional nurse. He also volunteered his time to mentor high school students. Howard, who weighed 308 pounds, didn't have a lot of free time; he had to exercise in the morning or not at all.

He began waking up a few minutes earlier each day to do his 8 Minutes in the Morning exercises. Being on my program, he lost more than 75 pounds, changed his diet, turned his bedroom into an exercise room, and began getting up at 4:30 A.M. to do his exercises, followed by 4 or more miles of powerwalking. "The morning exercises are great, and the effect really accumulates," Howard said. "For me, the morning exercise program creates wonderful results without struggle."

Without struggle!

Another one of my clients, Joseph Newsome, put it this way: "The morning exercises get my day started and leave me feeling great. My energy has risen to a level that I cannot ever remember having. I start my day feeling pumped up!"

Morning Benefits

When people ask me if they can do their 8 Minutes at any time of the day, I tell them that they will miss out on three major benefits. Exercising in the morning will:

• Boost your metabolism—BOOST!
• Let you maintain consistency—MAINTAIN!
• Allow you to enjoy your weight-loss journey—ENJOY!

When you first wake up in the morning, your metabolism is sluggish because it has slowed down during sleep. When you exercise, your metabolism increases. Thus, exercising in the morning enhances your metabolism when it's naturally the slowest. The bottom line is that physiologically, you burn more fat when you exercise in the morning, making better use of your exercise time.

Morning is the only time of day that most people can control. Later in the day, distractions will come up. Things that demand your time—including your spouse, your children, your job—will interrupt your schedule. You may plan to do your exercises during a lunch break, but a friend asks you to lunch and you think, "Okay, I'll do them after work." But after work, your 10-year-old asks for help with his homework. Then your husband wants to snuggle on the couch.

A 500-person study conducted at the Mollen Clinic in Phoenix showed that only 25 percent of evening exercisers consistently do their exercise routines, compared to 75 percent of morning exercisers. The bottom line is that when you commit to exercising in the morning, you bypass excuses and get the fat off faster. The clinic's founder, Art Mollen, D.O., says that "as the day goes on, people pull out the bow and arrows and hunt for excuses not to exercise—like having to work a bit later, run errands, or go out with friends."

In a study at the University of Leeds in England, researchers found that women who worked out in the morning reported less tension and greater feelings of contentment than those who didn't exercise in the morning. Exercising sends a signal to your pituitary gland to release endorphins, your body's

Frequently Asked Questions

What if my workouts take longer than 8 minutes?

Don't worry. Once you get the hang of the exercises and routine, they will go even faster. You should take about 1 minute to perform one set of 12 repetitions of an exercise. The key is to *immediately* move to the second exercise. Do this for a total of four sets, and you should be done in 8 minutes.

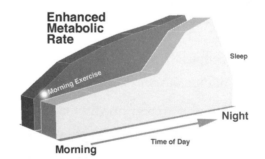

Though your metabolism naturally spikes sometime after midday, exercising first thing in the morning will increase it immediately so that you can reap the benefits all day long.

natural feel-good drug, first thing in the day. The more endorphins you have in your bloodstream, the better you feel. When you exercise in the morning, you will feel and handle yourself better no matter what happens in your day, whether it's getting stuck in a traffic jam, dealing with an annoying coworker, or tending to a sick child.

There are other benefits to morning exercise to consider. First, a study at Indiana University, in Bloomington, suggests that morning workouts reduce blood pressure. In fact, morning exercisers experienced an 8-point drop in systolic pressure (top number) that lasted 11 hours. Their diastolic pressure (bottom number) dropped 6 points for up to 4 hours after exercise. Evening exercisers showed no significant reductions.

There is some evidence, according to the American College of Sports Medicine, in Indianapolis, that confirms that hormonal responses to strength training are strongest in the morning. Resting levels of testosterone, the body's primary muscle-building hormone, are highest in the morning. In addition, following a bout of resistance training, testosterone elevations are more marked in the morning compared to the afternoon or early evening. This suggests that the muscle-building potential of strength training may be at its peak before noon.

The bottom line is that exercising is the ultimate endorphin booster and your ultimate advantage to enjoying your new lifestyle. You'll feel healthy after your morning sessions, which will help you focus on your Eat Fat to Get Fit eating plan and help motivate you each step of the way.

Sleep: Repair Muscles and Get Firmer

Most people have trouble waking up in the morning because they don't get enough sleep at night. On average, most people get at least an hour too little sleep on a regular basis.

In addition to diet and exercise, sleep is one of the most important components of a long and healthful life. If you get too little sleep, you eat more just to stay awake. Plus studies show that lack of sleep also can slow your metabolism, preventing your body from using glucose effectively.

Lack of sleep also affects your levels of leptin, the hormone that makes you feel full. When levels are low, you crave sweets such as candy, desserts, and even starches.

But the worst effects of sleep deprivation have to do with growth hormone levels. Growth hormone affects your body's proportion of fat to muscle as well as repairs muscles while you sleep. If you don't get enough sleep at night, your daily exercise session will feel harder than it should. You'll have a harder time building muscle and keeping fat at bay.

You have to promise yourself that you will really start going to bed earlier. It will help you wake up earlier and lose weight faster. It's that important to you.

Eat Fat to Get Fit

Bring Back the Joy of Eating and Lose More Weight

To get the results you want, you must combine your 8 Minutes in the Morning exercise routine with my Eat Fat to Get Fit Eating Card System. You heard right . . . eat fat! A simple little three-letter word, fat is too often overlooked when people are trying to lose weight. Most of us have been programmed to believe that all fats are bad and will only make us fatter. But we have been misled. It is essential for you to know that *eating a fat-free diet is the worst thing you can do when you want to lose weight!*

Fat

I have broken the program down into seven different food groups: Fat, Protein, Complex Carbohydrates, Dairy, Vegetables, Fruits, and Treats and Cravings. With each food group broken down, it is very simple to monitor what you eat if you follow the Eating Card System (see page 70). The Eating Cards will help you know that you have gotten all of the right foods in your body and the good and bad characteristics of each. The more you understand what you eat and why, the better choices you will make. (And, as always, you must drink you water—no less than eight glasses per day.)

Certain fats are considered "good" fats and, when eaten with your meals, are critical to maximizing your weight loss. There are three amazing ways that these good fats will help you lose weight. They:

• Are the ultimate appetite suppressant—SUPPRESS!
• Help unlock stored body fat—UNLOCK!
• Boost your body's metabolic rate, helping you to burn more body fat—BURN!

Think of it as a mantra: "Suppress, unlock, and burn!" (Like "Boost, maintain, and enjoy!" on page 43.) This is how you will Eat Fat to Get Fit. Read on to see why low-fat and nonfat diets are not the answer, then find out what the good fats are, how they work exactly, and where you can get them.

The Big Fat Misunderstanding

Over the past decade, fat has earned a bad reputation. Magazine articles, food marketers, and even weight-loss experts have told us that all fats are bad and that eating any type of fat will make *you* fat. This thinking promoted and perpetuated the no-fat craze, and food companies have made millions of dollars off it. Just visit the supermarket and look at all the fat-free versions of your favorite foods in one aisle after another.

Oddly enough, throughout this entire no-fat craze, people continued to get fatter. They bought up fat-free cookies, chips, and pastries but their waistlines expanded. How could that happen? For one, to make fat-free foods taste good, manufacturers had to add more sugar. Essentially, by the time they were done creating the fat-free version of the cookie or cheesecake, the product had just as many calories as the higher-fat version.

Scientists once thought that if you cut fat out of your diet, you would lose weight. They based this thinking on a number of factors, including that 1 gram of fat equals 9 calories, whereas 1 gram of carbohydrate or protein equals just 4. Coupled with that was the misconception that all dietary fat is converted to body fat more easily than carbohydrates or proteins. This led people to believe that they could only gain weight by eating fat, and that they could eat as much as they wanted all the time, as long as it was fat-free.

Avoid the Fat Trap

To avoid fattening, unhealthful fats, you need to understand what types of foods they hide in. Here are some examples for two specific types of bad fats.

Saturated fats. Found exclusively in high amounts in animal products such as beef, milk, cheese, lunchmeat, butter, and bacon. You can avoid these fats—and continue to eat animal products—if you:

• Choose lower-fat options such as white meat chicken and turkey without the skin, and reduced-fat dairy products. Even with red meat, look for the lowest-fat options (ground sirloin or round, sirloin steaks, reduced-fat lunchmeat, reduced-fat bacon and ham). I also recommend that you try soy versions of traditional meat—they taste great and are much more healthy.

• Watch your portion size. Think of meat and dairy products as condiments, not as your main course. Hold yourself to a 3- to 6-ounce serving of meat a day, roughly the size of one to two decks of cards. My Eating Card System will help you stay on track.

Trans fats. Also called hydrogenated fats, trans fats have no physical purpose in your body. They are a type of fat you could cut completely out of your diet and not have your body notice the difference. These fats are made when foods are processed, so they can be found in just about everything that has been boxed or changed from its natural state. Common trans fat culprits include biscuits, cakes, cinnamon buns, chips, crackers, doughnuts, muffins, pie crusts, many types of popcorn, and shortening.

The Fear of Fats

I'm sure most of you are thinking the same thing: "Wait a minute! If I include more fat in my diet, I am just going to get fatter!" Although fat does have nearly double the calories of carbohydrates and proteins, not all calories—and certainly not all fats—are created equally.

Some fats are not good for you and are converted to body fat faster, especially those that are saturated, hydrogenated, fried, or heat-processed. Found in red meat, butter, margarine, fried chicken, and doughnuts, these fats tend to trigger eating episodes. (Don't worry, you can still eat these foods. I will show you how.) If you've ever had one, you know exactly what I'm talking about. A coworker brings in a box of doughnuts. You decide that you'll have one to make her feel good. Suddenly, you've eaten not one but two doughnuts as well as a bag of chips.

Studies show that these types of fats are indeed addictive, making you want to eat more. They are also incredibly bad for your health. Saturated and hydrogenated fats have been linked to just about every health condition from heart disease to diabetes to cancer.

I do not recommend these fats in my Eat Fat to Get Fit program, but you can have them in moderation. More important, you will discover the good fats, the fats that I want you to incorporate into all your meals. These are called *omega fats*, and they'll help you get lean while making your food taste great.

What exactly are omega fats? They are sometimes called essential fatty acids (EFAs), because they are fats your body cannot make and must have for optimum performance. They are almost never stored as fat because they are used by your body in maintaining healthy cell membranes, brain function, healthy skin, strong hair, and strong nails and are directly related to thousands of life-sustaining metabolic functions.

Three of the most well-known and well-researched omega fats are the omega-3's, omega-6's, and omega-9's. Though omega-9 fats are not considered essential, they are still critical because they enhance the benefits of the omega-3's. I strongly recommend that you include all three types of fats in your meal plan.

So how do omega fats get you slim? As I shared with you at the beginning of this chapter, there are three amazing weight-loss benefits to using omega fats.

Suppress Appetite

Probably the most powerful benefit that omega fats give you is that they are the ultimate appetite suppressant. By adding omega fats to your foods or taking them with a meal, you will have a strong feeling of satiation, fullness, and satisfaction. Omega fats cause the stomach to retain food for a longer period of time as compared to no-fat or low-fat foods. That's because fats require greater digestive energy than proteins and carbohydrates. As a result, they are held in the stomach longer than other food sources, and they help to stimulate the release of cholecystokinin (CCK), a gut hormone that signals the brain to stop eating. According to studies done at Pennsylvania State University, in University Park, and Thomas Jefferson University–Jefferson Medical College, in Philadelphia, of all the nutrients you can eat, omega fats do the best job of promoting the feeling of fullness and satiety. In other words, you require smaller meals to make you feel satisfied, and you stay satisfied for longer periods of time—up to 6 hours.

My good friend Jade Beutler, author of two wonderful books, *Understanding Fats and Oils* and *Flax for Life*, shared with me a great metaphor that I will never forget. He says that when you eat omega fats, you can think of yourself as a superefficient automobile getting 30 miles per gallon of gas; as opposed to a gas hog that is getting 10 miles per gallon (when you eat fat-free). The gas hog uses more fuel more quickly and therefore has to stop more frequently at the pump (or refrigerator) to fill up. But by eating your meals with omega fats, you automatically get better "gas mileage."

And that's the ticket. You will feel fuller longer and not experience hunger pangs or the desire to snack between meals.

Eat Fat to Get Fit Quick Reference Chart

Omega-3. Get it from liquid flax oil (make this the primary fat that you add to your meals). Use it on salads or bread, and add it to soups (after cooking) and yogurt. Do not cook with this fat.

Omega-6. You get omega-6's from prepackaged foods like chips and store-bought foods. You get enough of this fat, so avoid adding it to your meals.

Omega-9. Olive oil, avocados, peanuts, almonds, and macadamia nuts all include omega-9 fats. It's the second-best oil to add to your meals because it enhances your use of omega-3 fat. Olive oil should be your number-one cooking fat. When eating out in restaurants, ask for olive oil to use on your salad instead of dressing, and dip your bread into it instead of using butter.

Unlock Stored Body Fat

Eating the right amounts of omega fats helps to *unlock stored body fat so that you can better use it as energy*. Omega fat balances your body's ratio of insulin to glucagon. When you eat sugary foods, your body secretes the hormone insulin to remove the excess sugar from your body. When you eat excessively sugary meals, your body releases too much insulin, blocking the critical pancreatic hormone glucagon from operating effectively within your body. Glucagon is a key hormone that enables your body to burn its stores of body fat. A diet rich in omega fats helps balance your insulin levels so that glucagon can be released to unlock your body's fat-storage banks and begin converting unwanted body fat into energy.

Burn Body Fat

Omega fats boost your body's metabolic rate, which in turn helps you burn more body fat! No other fat on Earth will do this. Your metabolic rate will increase in two natural and healthy ways. Your body will immediately utilize the omega fats to maintain the integrity and function of your body's 75 trillion cell membranes. Having healthier cell membranes means that you improve the "vehicles" that transport oxygen, one of the key elements in everyday fat burning. The more oxygen you have available, the easier it is for your lean muscle tissue to convert body fat into the energy it needs to sustain itself.

The body fat you want to burn, called white fat, lies near the top of your skin. There is another type of fat, called brown fat, that lies deep within your body and surrounds your vital organs—your heart, kidneys, and adrenal glands. It also cushions your spinal column as well as your neck and major thoracic blood vessels.

By *activating* your brown fat, your body will burn more calories for heat rather than retaining those calories for future use. Brown fat is not a storage fat like white fat, but rather a calorie-burning engine. Ann Louise Gittleman, M.S., C.N.S., one of the foremost nutritionists in the United States, explains that "although brown fat makes up 10 percent or less of total body fat, it is responsible for 25 percent of all the fat calories burned by all the other body tissues." So having a second type of fat-burning furnace is almost like having more lean muscle tissue!

Still not convinced that you can Eat Fat to Get Fit . . . that you will lose weight and look great? Just read what a few of my clients have to say about adding omega fats to their diets.

• "I spent months eating low-fat foods and doing 60 minutes of high-impact aerobics everyday and got nowhere. When I was unable to fit into my pre-pregnancy clothes after 2 years, I became depressed," says Stephanie Donald. "When I started to Eat Fat to Get Fit, I weighed 162 pounds and had a 31-inch waist. After 8 weeks, I had lost 14 pounds and 2 inches from my waist!"

• "I do not feel like I'm in food prison with many restrictions and limitations," says former emotional eater Howard Joseph.

• "Adding omega fats to my diet made me feel satisfied," says Amber Dunlap. "I don't feel moody as I did with other diets that I've tried. I really like that I am eating enough for my body, and I can feel the difference. The fat is melting off! This is the easiest weight I have ever lost!"

Good for Your Health, Too

The Eat Fat to Get Fit program not only helps you shed the pounds but also helps you live longer. The unappreciated good guys for a number of years, omega fats have only relatively recently received the respect they deserve. Quite a bit of research has been done that supports the

Omega Fats = Good Fats

Though any fat can help satisfy your appetite or even release stored body fat, omega fats, particularly omega-3's, offer a number of uniquely wonderful benefits.

• They cannot ever be converted into the "bad" saturated fats. This is important because excessive intake of saturated fat is closely linked to obesity, cancer, heart disease, stroke, and premature death. Hundreds of research studies show that omega fats can actually help prevent all these things, plus certain types of diabetes.
• In women, omega fats have been shown to help ease premenstrual syndrome and postmenopausal discomforts.
• In men, omega fats have been shown to improve sex drive.

idea of using omega fats to help you reach your weight-loss goal as well as improve your overall health.

• A study completed in the United Kingdom found that supplementing with omega fats—not saturated fats or even polyunsaturated fats—changed the composition of joint cartilage, reducing the pain and inflammation associated with various types of arthritis. Another study found that patients who took omega fat supplements were able to completely stop taking their anti-inflammatory painkillers for arthritic disease.

• A study from Korea found that people who eat more omega fats on a daily basis experience a lower risk of prostate cancer and prostate inflammation. Numerous other studies have shown a decreased risk for other types of cancers as well.

• A study done in the Netherlands found that supplementing with omega fats reduced some of the intestinal inflammation associated with Crohn's disease. Many other studies have shown that diets high in omega fats reduce all sorts of gastrointestinal problems, from chronic diarrhea to chronic constipation.

• Research strongly shows that increasing the omega fats in your diet while simultaneously decreasing the saturated and trans fats can boost immunity, regulate blood sugar, prevent diabetes, reduce heart disease and stroke, treat asthma, lift depression, prevent Alzheimer's disease, and, of course, promote weight loss.

Here are some tips to help you get more healthy good fats into your diet.

• Although cold-water fish such as salmon and mackerel are higher in protein than they are in fat, they do contain enough omega-3 fatty acids to deserve a mention here.

Since fish is not a superconcentrated source of omega fats, you will only check off Protein boxes and *not* check off a Fat box on your Eating Cards. It is great for lunch or dinner.

• If you like butter, you can make your own healthy butter substitute. Pour extra-virgin olive oil (omega-9 fat) into a plastic airtight container and then cover. Refrigerate it overnight to harden it. Then you can spread it just as you would butter!

• Going nuts for a great midday snack? Try almonds. These healthful nuts make a perfect snack because they are packed full of omega-9 fats and will help you burn fat while satisfying your midday hunger pangs. Other omega-packed nuts include hazelnuts, pecans, macadamia nuts, and pistachios.

• Eat avocados. These green, pear-shaped foods taste so delicious that it's hard to believe they are also good for you. Avocado makes a great spread on whole wheat toast instead of sugary jam. It's even great to add to any salad. A ripe avocado is slightly soft—not hard—to your touch.

• Use olive oil in place of salad dressing on your veggies or when you don't have flax oil available.

The Best Slimming Omega Source

The best omega fat source for weight loss is one that is the richest in omega-3 fat. Why omega-3, and not omega-6 or omega-9? Omega-3 fat is the least *saturated fat*—the most pliable and nonsolid. That means that omega-3 fat is the body's top choice for maintaining everything from healthy cell membranes to brain function. When your body uses the omega-3 fats for these types of necessary bodily functions, there is literally no more of it left to be stored on your body as body fat.

Why does your body better utilize a fat that is the least saturated, such as omega-3 fat rather than a fat that is more saturated? Imagine that you are part of the body's "maintenance team" and you are assigned to maintain a cell membrane. Your goal is to keep the cell membrane healthy and alive. To do this, you need some building materials, and one of them is fat. The worst kind of fat you could use is one that is solid and hard, otherwise

Finding the Friendly Fats

Where is the best place to find omega-3 fat? Check out the chart below to see which source is the best choice. Fresh flax oil is the winner, with a whopping 57 percent of the precious omega-3 fat.

	Monounsaturated Omega-9	Polyunsaturated Omega-6	Polyunsaturated Omega-3
Saturated Fat	Oleic Acid	Linoleic Acid	Alpha-Linolenic Acid

Saturated	Monounsaturated	Polyunsaturated Omega-6	Polyunsaturated Omega-3	Source
9%		65%	26%	Almond
6%		64%	30%	Apricot Kernel
20%		70%	10%	Avocado
6%		60%	24%	10%	Corn
13%	27%		60%	Canola
9%	16%	18%	57%	Fresh Flax (Linseed)
12%	17%		71%	Grape Seed
10%		82%	8%	Olive
19%		51%	30%	Peanut
9%	34%	42%	15%	Pumpkinseed
8%	13%		79%	Safflower
13%	46%		41%	Sesame
14%	28%	50%	8%	Soy
12%	19%		69%	Sunflower
16%	28%	51%	5%	Walnut

SOURCE: NatureMed Research, Inc.

known as a saturated fat. If you used these hard, sticky, gluelike saturated fats, the cell membrane would soon become stiff, too. That means the cell itself would get less oxygen, age faster, and die faster. This is not good because you not only age faster but also you are more susceptible to things like cancer and heart disease. If you had your choice, you would select the least saturated fat possible, and that would be an omega-3 fat, followed by the omega-6 and the omega-9, respectively. Just remember, the lower the number, the better the fat is for you. The higher the number, the more saturated it is. For a comparison of the omega fats, see "Finding the Friendly Fats."

Fabulous Flax

Flax oil is the ideal weight-loss fat because it is the richest source of omega-3 fats. Plus, it has the ideal amount of omega-6 and omega-9. Recall that omega-6 fat is the only

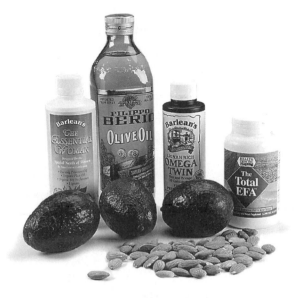

Eating more omega fats will help you eat less, enjoy your food, boost your metabolism, prevent disease, and feel happier.

other fat that your body cannot make. You get omega-6's from things like safflower, soybean, or corn oils, which are fats that are used in many pre-packaged foods. So, most of us are getting plenty of omega-6 already. What you need to focus on is getting more omega-3's into your diet with flax. Flax also contains omega-9, and though it's not essential, the positive effects of the Mediterranean diet are largely attributed to omega-9 fatty acids. The bottom line is that flax oil has a perfect blend of all three omega fats to help you lose the weight!

Flax oil comes from flaxseeds, also called linseeds. I recommend that you buy flax in liquid form because it is the most efficient. The oil is made by cold-pressing thousands of seeds to extract the oil. The oil is immediately refrigerated to preserve its freshness. You can use the liquid form directly on your foods, and this is where the flavor and fun starts. Think of it as a great flavor-enhancing condiment you can use with all your meals. I use it during breakfast on toast, at lunch I put it on my salad, and at dinner, I use it on my brown rice or steamed veggies. Liquid flax oil can be found in all health food stores. And for those of you who travel or just don't care for the taste of fat, you can get flax oil in capsule forms too.

Just how important is supplementing your diet with liquid flax oil? I am such a big believer in the weight-loss power of flax, I wanted to make sure that all my clients would be able to conveniently find the finest

How to "Flaxsize" Your Meals

Here are a few tips to easily add flax oil into your meals. If you want to share your great ideas for getting more flax into your diet, e-mail them to flaxsize@jorgecruise.com.

- Instead of a sugary jam spread on your toast in the morning, use flax oil (pretend it is melted butter). It will make your toast taste better and you will feel fuller longer.

- Use a teaspoon of flax oil at lunch or dinner in place of salad dressing on your veggies.

- Eat a nonfat yogurt or soy yogurt mixed with a teaspoon of flax oil 1 hour before dinner to keep you from overeating.

- Make soup a more filling, fat-burning friend by adding a teaspoon of flax oil after cooking. It will activate your metabolism and improve the flavor of the soup.

grade of flax possible at the best price. So I created my own brand of liquid flax oil and capsules synergized with a proprietary blend of enzymes and antioxidants. Virtually all the people in the success stories in this book used it. I personally use the liquid version every day and when I travel, I use the capsules. (For more information on *Jorge Cruise's Flax Oil*, visit www.jorgecruise.com/flax.)

How Much Fat

I don't want you to think that you can eat only omega fats on this program. You can still enjoy a variety of fats with your meals, even saturated fats like butter, and you can still use corn oil or whatever other oils you like—just use them in moderation. A complete list of all the fats you can use on this program appears on page 211.

The amount of fat you need depends on your current weight and caloric needs. Don't worry. You don't need to spend any time with a calculator and chart to figure out how much fat to eat in a day. I've done all the work for you. As long as you use your Eating Card

System, you will automatically eat the right amount and right types of fat at every meal.

I've also assembled an easy-to-use general Food List (see page 211) that will help you make smart choices and check off the correct boxes with your Eating Card System (see page 70).

I've also assembled an easy-to-use general Food List (see page 211) that will help you make smart choices and check off the correct boxes with your Eating Card System (see page 70).

The Right Portions

To check off the right number of boxes in your Eating Card System, you have to know how much you are eating. But you don't need to measure and weigh everything you eat. Here are some simple examples of how to approximately gauge your food portions by comparing them to the size of parts of your hand.

Thumb tip: 1 box of olive oil, flax oil, or avocado

Fist: 1 box of green vegetables, grains, or whole fruit

Cupped hand: 1 box of dairy

Palm of hand (excluding fingers and thumb): 3 boxes of protein

Protein

Have you ever lost a significant amount of weight on a diet, only to plateau well before you reached your goal? That's probably because you weren't eating enough protein. Sometimes eating more helps you lose more weight.

Protein is your body's building material. You need to eat protein to provide your body with the materials it needs to build, repair, and maintain your lean muscle tissue. That's incredibly important because without enough dietary protein, all of your 8 Minutes in the Morning moves will be for naught. And over half of your body weight is made up of protein. This includes not only muscle tissue but also hair, skin, nails, blood, hormones, enzymes, brain cells, and much more.

When you don't eat enough protein, your body actually starts to break down and recycle existing body protein (such as lean muscle) to supply your body with the amino acids that your diet is lacking. When this protein breakdown occurs, you sacrifice muscle (your fat-burning machine) and your metabolism slows down. As a result, you burn less body fat.

Protein is important, but don't go overboard. You've probably heard about—and may have even tried—one of the popular high-protein diets. When I interviewed best-selling author Andrew Weil, M.D., for my FitNow.com online television show, he shared with me what's wrong with these diets: They work for weight loss—temporarily—because you're eating more protein than your body needs to repair tissue, and your body burns the excess as fuel. Unfortunately, protein is a "dirty" source of fuel because it contains nitrogen. Instead of producing just carbon dioxide and water, protein produces nitrogenous residues, which are toxic. Your body must pump a lot of water into the urinary tract to flush the toxic nitrogen out. In other words, much of the "weight loss" from high-protein diets is simply water loss. While this is going on, you're also losing minerals from your body, including calcium from your bones.

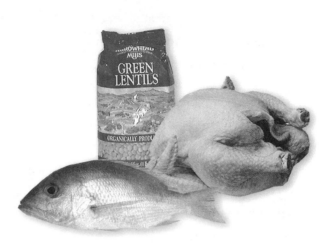

Eating more of the right types of protein will help you build calorie-hungry muscle, boost your metabolism, and feel less hungry.

To eat the right amount of protein, all you need to do is follow your Eating Card System and consult the Food List on page 211 for the best sources.

Besides getting protein in the right amounts, you also want to focus on the right types. Some types of protein—especially the type found in animal products—contain a high amount of saturated fat, which can not only hinder your weight-loss efforts but also destroy your health. Focus on high-quality protein sources like fish, skinless white-meat chicken, turkey meat, soy products, egg whites, legumes, and beans.

Soybeans are a quality protein source that is naturally low in saturated fat. If you're a vegetarian, eating soy is the best way to ensure that you consume all of the amino acids you need. Even if you're not a vegetarian, I recommend adding soy to your diet because it has been shown to reduce heart disease, cancer, osteoporosis, menopausal symptoms, and more. You'll find it in veggie versions of burgers, hot dogs, lunchmeats, and cheeses as well as in tofu, miso, soy milk, and soy nuts. Tofu is a great meat extender. Mix it with meat or cheese to lower the saturated fat in your recipes.

When you have a hankering for red meat, go ahead and have it, but choose lean sirloin or round cuts, eat a small portion, and trim off any visible fat. Limit your red meat consumption to no more than twice a week. Beef comes marbled with nonessential fat that is mostly saturated. It is the worst animal fat in terms of chemical composition, containing 51 percent saturated fatty acids (SFAs). In comparison, pig lard, still very bad, has 41 percent SFAs.

Complex Carbohydrates

My Eat Fat to Get Fit program includes carbohydrates because they play a critical role in achieving fat loss. You read it right: Carbohydrates can be used to get you lean. The key is to avoid simple carbohydrates that are high on the glycemic index, which rates how fast a particular food turns into glucose (blood sugar), and eat complex carbohydrates that are much lower on the index. The higher the number, the faster it turns into glucose. Simple carbohydrates such as processed white bread and rice release quickly. Complex carbohydrates, on the other hand, are usually whole grain and unprocessed.

How does avoiding simple carbohydrates help you burn body fat? When your insulin is balanced, more of the hormone glucagon is available to help unlock body fat stores. You can help balance insulin levels further by avoiding the foods that drastically increase insulin levels: simple carbohydrates.

Simple vs. Complex

Simple carbohydrates not only prevent you from burning pre-existing body fat but also encourage you to gain more body fat. When you eat a large meal that is made from simple carbohydrates, you are left with an immediate abundance of glucose, more than your body could ever need or use. Some of the glucose that is not used right away by your muscles is stored in your liver and muscles as glycogen (stored blood sugar). The rest is converted and stored as body fat. This is why you can remain overweight even though you are eating low-fat or nonfat foods.

The solution is to eat complex carbohydrates, which provide you with just the right amount of energy while burning excess body fat. Imagine that you're starting a campfire. You would light the big logs by using lighter fluid or kindling. That's exactly how complex carbohydrates work in your body. Instead of wood, it's body fat. By trickling in small amounts of complex carbohydrates, the fat will burn steadily for a long time. If you pour too much lighter fluid (simple carbohydrates) on at one time, you get a flash fire that flares quickly and then burns out almost immediately.

Unlike simple carbohydrates, complex carbohydrates are not rapidly released into your bloodstream because of their complex molecular structure. This means that complex carbohydrates never overwhelm your body with sugar rushes because they take more time to break down. They provide the ideal amounts of time-released sugar to burn fat. This allows your body to use body fat as its primary fuel.

To find out which foods are complex carbohydrates and which are simple carbohydrates, consult the Food List on page 211. But you can also use this simple rule of thumb: The more "whole" or natural a food is, the more likely it is to be complex.

Whole Grains

Whole grains—those that contain their outer shells—are more complex than refined grains, which have been stripped of their outer coatings. In other words, slow-cooking, whole grain oats are better than instant oats, brown rice is better than white rice, whole grain bread is better than white bread, and whole grain pasta is better than regular pasta. Another good rule of thumb is to check the fiber content. Foods that are higher in fiber—with at least 3 or more grams—tend to be more "whole" than foods that lack fiber.

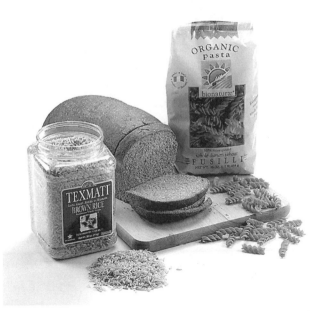

Eating more of the right types of carbohydrates will help you burn more body fat, balance insulin levels, feel less hungry, and prevent disease.

Whole grains are also incredibly good for your health. That outer covering of the grain contains disease-fighting fiber and important phytochemicals. Here are some ways to add different grains to your diet.

• Treat yourself to whole grain breads from an old-fashioned bakery.

• The slower oatmeal cooks, the more "whole" it is. Irish oatmeal (also called Scotch or steel-cut oats) is your best source of whole grains. If you don't have time to wait for it to cook on the stove, add it to other recipes, such as meat loaf and stuffing.

• Breakfast cereals are a great source of whole grains *if* you buy the right kind. The high-sugar, overly processed "kiddie" cereals are not going to cut it. The better breakfast cereals, such as Uncle Sam (visit www.jorgecruise.com/unclesam for more information on this cereal), contain at least 3 grams of fiber and less than 1 gram of total fat.

• High in protein and free from gluten, quinoa is a great grain substitute if you are allergic to wheat. It also contains lots of calcium, iron, fiber, B vitamins, vitamin E, and folate. It is one of my favorite hot cereals. Add quinoa to soups, stews, and cold salads.

Dairy

Dairy is supposed to be good for you—its main selling point being that it's high in calcium—but what if you are allergic to it? It was after I read *Eating Well for Optimum Health*, an amazing book by Dr. Andrew Weil, that my viewpoint on dairy changed. The protein found in dairy products, called casein, is a known allergen that can cause asthma and sinus problems and can be an irritant to your immune system. Casein has been shown to trigger an autoimmune reaction that destroys insulin-producing cells in the pancreas. That can lead to juvenile diabetes. And digestion of lactose (the sugar in milk) requires the enzyme lactase, which many adults lack. This can cause major digestive distress.

You can get the calcium you need from fortified soy products such as soy milk and soy cheese instead. These are both delicious and healthy alternatives that I use every day. You can also get calcium from fortified juice. Most people don't realize that all green plants have high levels of calcium, particularly broccoli, collards, and kale. And you can always take a calcium supplement. If you don't have asthma, chronic allergies, hay fever, or sinus problems, you can eat traditional dairy products in moderation; I use dairy mostly as a condiment. Just make sure you use products that are low-fat or made from nonfat milk.

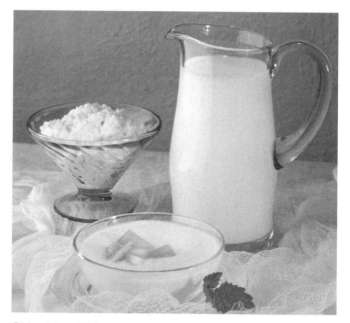

Select healthier versions of dairy, such as soy, to support your weight loss by reducing sinus problems so that you get more oxygen to burn body fat, boosting your immune system, and helping eliminate asthma.

Vegetables

Although vegetables are a type of carbohydrate, I've grouped them in their own category because of their unique beneficial effects on fat loss. Vegetables have a very high water content, which means that they are also very high in oxygen. In order for your lean muscle tissue to burn fat, it needs oxygen to help convert the fat into energy. When you eat vegetables, you will flood your body with water, which will dramatically increase your oxygen levels, improving your metabolism.

Vegetables are high in fiber and, ounce for ounce, are probably the most filling low-calorie food you can eat. And since vegetables need to be chewed more and take longer to consume, your brain has time to realize that you are eating and turns off the "hunger switch" sooner. Once in your stomach, that fiber takes up a lot of space, making you feel full.

Most vegetables are also very low in simple sugars. Vegetables have almost no calories. This means you can literally eat them to your heart's content and not put on excess body fat. For example, to consume a paltry 20 calories, you would have to eat half a cucumber, 4 cups of a butterhead lettuce such as Bibb or Boston, or 1 cup of radish slices.

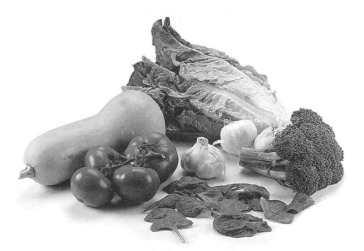

Vegetables are high in water and oxygen, which improves your metabolism; high in fiber, which fills you up; low in simple sugars, which encourages the release of glucagon; low in calories; and high in phytochemicals, which boosts your overall immunity.

Besides promoting weight loss, vegetables are superfoods when it comes to your health. They are an important source of vitamins and minerals, and research has shown that brightly colored vegetables contain substances called phytochemicals that form the plant's immune system. These phytochemicals also act to keep the human immune system strong. In just one serving of green

Frequently Asked Questions

What's your favorite way to make vegetables more exciting to eat?

One of my clients shared this incredibly simple recipe for a tasty veggie dressing. Combine the juice from half of a lemon with 1 teaspoon flax oil (1 Fat box) and one minced garlic clove. Pour over your salad or crudités and enjoy. For more great food ideas, see page 227 and visit www.jorgecruise.com.

vegetables, more than 100 different phytochemicals may be present to help ward off disease. Think about it. If you are sick less often, you will have more energy to do the things you love, including sticking to your 8 Minutes in the Morning program.

You can eat almost all vegetables in unlimited amounts on this program—that's how low in calories and how good for you they are. Only a few vegetables—especially potatoes and other root vegetables that are high in starch—contain more calories, and therefore can not be eaten with abandon.

Many people are out of the habit of eating vegetables. You want to eat as many servings of green vegetables as you can, particularly when you have a mood-related craving or feel hungry for no apparent reason. See page 227 for some recipes for all-you-can-eat green vegetables.

Fruits

You've probably been told that fruit is good for you. But that's true only if you're not trying to lose weight. While fruit does contain a wealth of beneficial nutrients that help your body fight off disease, it also contains high amounts of simple sugars.

Fruit, especially tropical fruit, is high on the glycemic index. Your body breaks it down and burns it quickly, spiking your insulin levels. High insulin levels block the hormone glucagon, hindering the fat-burning process.

Compared to green vegetables, fruit contains quite a few calories. One banana contains 100 calories, and ½ cup of fruit salad contains 110. Compare that to ½ cup of asparagus or ½ cup of broccoli for only 22 calories.

Fruit is good for you in other ways, so don't cut it completely out of your diet. I suggest holding yourself to only one serving a day, while pumping up your vegetable servings to six or more. Lemons and limes are the exception; feel free to use them

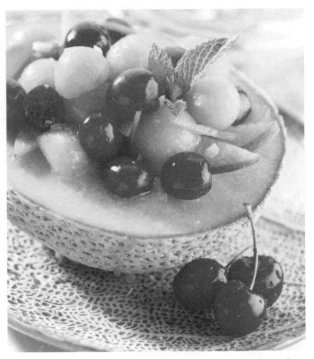

Limiting yourself to just one serving of fruit a day will lower your consumption of simple sugars, keep your insulin levels steady, and lower your calorie intake.

as much as you want. (I love to use lemon or lime in my water every day to help cleanse my body.)

If you love fruit and can't bear the thought of eating only one piece a day, cut your serving in half so that you can eat a small serving of fruit early in the day and another serving later on.

Treats and Cravings

No food is a bad food. Sure, some foods are a lot better for you than others, but I don't put any food on the "do not ever eat" list. That just sets you up for bingeing—as soon as you tell yourself that you are not allowed to eat something ever again, you want that food all the more. The foods in my Treats and Cravings category may not be the best foods for your health, but if you love them, you have to find a way to work them into your Eat Fat to Get Fit program.

Consult the Food List on page 211. I list 40 of the most highly craved foods, from ice cream to animal crackers, how much of them you can have, and how many boxes to check off on your Eating Cards. As long as you hold yourself to a small serving size, you can eat whatever food you want. If you want to go hog wild on a large-size dessert, make the bulk of your main meal extremely healthy, low-calorie greens. You must still follow your Eating Card System, and once you check off all the boxes, you're done eating for the day.

To prevent yourself from overdoing it with Treats and Cravings, heed the following advice when you feel a craving coming on.

Wait 10 minutes before indulging. Most cravings last only about 10 minutes and then subside. Cravings often are your body's cries for water and oxygen. So during those 10 minutes, drink a glass of water with lemon and take a few deep breaths. By giving your body these things, you can get through a craving

Frequently Asked Questions

I really love fruit, so it's been tough for me to eat it only once a day over the past 4 weeks. Once I reach my goal, may I add more fruit servings to my food plan?

You can eat more fruit as long as you substitute another food in its place. The best strategy is to substitute two Treats and Cravings for every extra serving of fruit. But first, try splitting the one serving in half so that you can eat fruit twice a day.

just fine. You might even want to change activities to clear your mind. Go for a walk or take a shower.

Brush your teeth and tongue. This will get the taste of food out of your mouth and ruin the idea of eating something indulgent like fudge. (Chocolate and toothpaste simply don't go together.) Food is less tempting when your mouth feels clean.

Never skip a meal. If you skip a meal, you will feel ravenous and out of control. Be sure to enjoy every one of your meals.

Water

Although not a food category, water is an essential component of my Eat Fat to Get Fit program. The typical person needs eight 8-ounce glasses of water a day just for basic maintenance. Most people drink only four to five glasses.

Your body needs water for everything from maintaining blood volume to skin health to toxin release. Without it, your energy level plummets, you get headaches, and you simply don't feel like exercising. Even mild dehydration (if you feel thirsty, you're already dehydrated) can make you feel tired. That's because the electrical and chemical signals in your brain ride on water. Dehydration also lowers your blood volume, making your heart pump harder to move blood throughout your body. That tires you out, too. Feeling tired means you won't have the energy to exercise, and you'll burn fewer calories.

Water as Food

Water takes up room in your stomach, making you feel full. That means you eat less and feel less hungry. At parties, keep a glass of water in your hand and sip it instead of grabbing a high-

Using the Eating Card System

The secret to the eating part of my program is eating the right amount of fat with each meal and monitoring your total food intake. You will do this with your Eating Card System.

Each Eating Card is made up a series of boxes that represent one selection from the food group. There are seven food groups in my Eat Fat to Get Fit eating plan:

1. Fats
2. Proteins
3. Complex Carbohydrates
4. Dairy
5. Vegetables
6. Fruits
7. Treats and Cravings

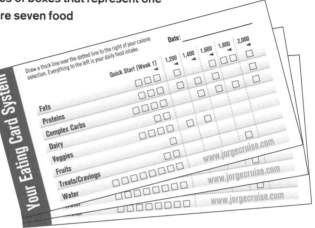

A compete list of all recommended foods from each food group is gathered in the Food List on page 211. Each time you eat one portion of food, cross off that box on the card with an X. If you eat three portions, you need to cross off three boxes.

Every time you sit down for a meal or snack, first go to the Food List and decide what you want to eat. Then look at how many boxes that food item uses. Each box equals one portion. The Food List indicates that ½ cup cooked pasta is one portion. Therefore, 1 cup of cooked pasta would equal two portions; you would check off 2 Complex Carbohydrate boxes. There is also a place on your card to check off eight daily glasses of water. Be sure to drink all of them.

When you finish crossing off all the boxes, you are finished eating for the day. The key is to make sure to eat all the food on your daily Eating Card. Some people think that they can hurry weight loss along by eating even less food than they are allowed on the card. That's dangerous because eating less will generate weight loss from muscle tissue, not just body fat. You must eat all of your food.

If you're still hungry after crossing off all of your boxes, refer to the Food List for the vegetables that you can eat without limit.

About the Cards

You'll see that I've included master Eating Cards on page 234. The Eating Cards are designed to be photocopied, ideally onto card stock. There are two of the same cards on the page. Make four copies, which gives you enough cards for 7 days plus an extra card. After you photocopy them, cut the cards down the middle and stack them. You can also staple them together to make a booklet. This is now your eating guide for the week. Take it with you everywhere you go. Imagine it's an eating "checkbook."

The First Week

For the first week, you will use the Quick Start portion of the Eating Card no matter what your current weight or goal. It's an eating plan that will cleanse your body and help you break your poor eating habits (see A Week of Eating Fat to Get Fit on page 219). It is essential that you follow it precisely. Look at it as a special time to start fresh. After the first week, you will feel great physically. So, to start, draw a thick line over the dotted line to the right of the Quick Start section. All the boxes to the left of this line represent how much you will eat each day of Week 1.

Weeks 2, 3, 4, and Beyond

For the remainder of the program, select the calorie intake that is right for you. How do you know which to use after Week 1?

Your Current Weight (lb)	Calories for Women	Calories for Men
Under 150	1,200	1,400
150–199	1,400	1,600
200–49	1,600	1,800
250–99	2,000	2,000
300+	For every 50 pounds above 300, add 1 Complex Carbohydrate selection and 1 Protein selection to the 2,000-Calorie section	For every 50 pounds above 300, add 1 Complex Carbohydrate selection and 1 Protein selection to the 2,000-Calorie section

For now, you will be using your gender and current weight as a guide. As your weight goes down, you will move to the next calorie selection to continue your fat burning. For example, if you are a woman who weighs 190 pounds, you will use the 1,400 Calories section. When you reach 149 pounds, you will change to the 1,200 Calories section. If you weigh more than 300 pounds, you will need additional calories as described in the chart.

Get a pen and draw a thick line over the dotted line to the right of your calorie selection. Everything to the left is your ideal daily food intake.

calorie mixed drink or reaching for the chips. And research shows that many people mistake thirst for hunger, so it's not a bad idea to gulp a glass of water every time you feel a craving, and then decide if you truly *need* to eat.

Of all the ways you can get fluid into your body, drinking water is the best because it has no calories. Zero. If you don't stick to water, your liquid calories can really add up. For example, just ½ cup of fruit juice contains 45 to 80 calories. And most people drink a lot more than ½ cup. A typical bottle of fruit juice drink can contain 150 calories or more. The café latte from your favorite coffeeshop chain can contain a whopping 320 calories. And that 32-ounce cola that you down at the movie theater contains more than 400 calories.

Eating Fit at Restaurants

Eating out is one of the scariest prospects that dieters face. There are so many tempting sights and smells. But you can eat out—in fact, you can eat anywhere—and still stick to your Eat Fat to Get Fit plan. Just follow these tips:

• Think of your Eating Card the same way you do your credit card: Never leave home without it.

• Know that you are the one who is paying the bill and that you are the one in charge. Look at the menu, ask questions, and make substitutions when necessary.

• Ask for dressings and sauces to be served on the side.

• When your plate arrives, portion your food *before* you start to eat. Ask for the rest to be wrapped immediately.

• Use extra-virgin olive oil instead of butter.

• Don't forget to eyeball your portion sizes; most restaurants are notorious for overfeeding people.

• Avoid all-you-can-eat buffets.

• Get a salad or vegetables instead of french fries.

• Know that a typical restaurant portion of meat is 9 to 12 ounces. Don't get carried away.

• Don't eat from anyone else's plate; that counts, too.

"Diet" drinks are a little better. Just limit yourself to two a day. (See page 218).

The worst slimming drink is alcohol; avoid it if you want to lose weight. It is very high in calories—almost equal to fat calories. If you do have an alcoholic drink, check off 2 Fat boxes on your Eating Cards, as specified for each amount. Drinking beer will require that you also check off 1 Complex Carbohydrate box.

Tips for Switching

It's easy to tell you all the things that are wrong with fruit drinks, coffee, diet drinks, and alcohol. It's another thing for you to just switch to drinking water all the time. Here are some tips to help you make the transition.

Create a concoction. If you don't like the taste of plain water, jazz it up. Try a sparkling water such as Perrier. Pour it into a glass and add some taste with a squeeze of juice from a lemon, lime, orange, or all three.

Limit yourself to two or fewer caffeinated drinks a day. I'm not going to make you give up your caffeine fix. But if you're the type of person who drinks diet soda from the moment you roll out of bed until the end of the workday, you need to cut back to only two of these drinks a day.

Make smarter choices. You can continue to have those wonderfully delicious coffee drinks if you will make a few simple switches. First, opt for cappuccino. Because they are made with more bubbles, cappuccinos naturally contain fewer calories than lattes and other coffee drinks. Also, order your cappuccino made with fat-free milk, which will bring your count down to only about 80 calories. And try soy cappuccino, which will give you a dose of healthy protein, making those calories more worthwhile. As for fruit juices, choose lower-calorie tomato juice and cranberry juice (with no sugar added). Mix higher-calorie juices with water to lower the calorie count even farther.

I like sugar in my iced tea. What should I do?

If you like your tea and coffee sweet, I recommend an herbal substitute called stevia. It is a great natural sweetener that will support your weight-loss goal; it can be found at almost all health food stores.

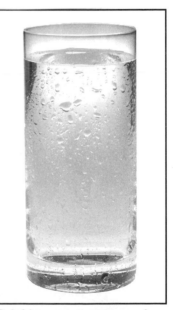

Drinking more water and fewer liquid calories will suppress your hunger, lower your calorie intake, cleanse your body, and give you more energy.

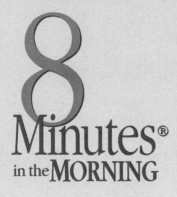

PART THREE

The Program

CHAPTER 7

4 Weeks to a New You

Putting Jorge's Plan into Action

I t's time for us to start training to-gether every day for the next 4 weeks. Everything you will need to achieve success will be right here. Each day of this 28-day pro-gram, you will take three simple steps:

1. Read Your Wake-Up Talk found on the first page of each day of the program. These talks will keep you energized and mo-tivated during the next 4 weeks and will help you get fit from the inside out. Never skip them; they're important.

2. Perform the two Today's Moves training exercises included within each

Warmup and Cooldown

Start your session with a short warmup to increase the temperature of your body and your joints. When your joints are cold, the fluid inside is thicker, making your joints feel stiff. Save stretching until after strength training to avoid muscle pulls and injuries. As with the rest of the 8 Minutes in the Morning program, your warm-up is simple.

Jog in place. Make sure to move both your arms and legs. How fast should you move? On a scale from 1 to 10, shoot for a 4 or 5, which is 40 to 50 percent of your maximum heart rate.

Cool down with a quick full-body stretching routine. This will increase your range of motion so you stay flexible and avoid injuries.

Sky-Reaching Pose: Stand tall and reach with both hands toward the sky. Reach as high as you comfortably can. Feel the stretch lengthening your spine, bringing more range of motion to your joints. Breathe deeply through your nose. Hold for 10 seconds to 1 minute.

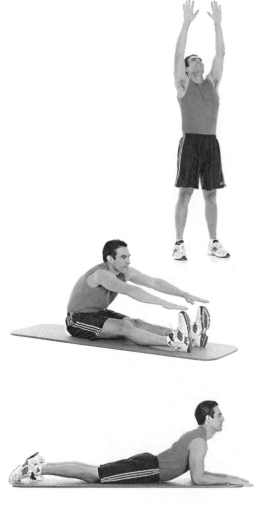

Hurdler's Stretch: Sit on a mat on the floor with your legs extended in front of you. Keeping your back flat, gently bend forward from the hips and reach as far as you can toward your toes. If possible, pull your toes back slightly toward your upper body. Hold for 10 seconds to 1 minute.

Cobra Stretch: Lie on a mat on your belly with your palms flat on the ground next to your shoulders and your legs just slightly less than shoulder-width apart. Your feet should be resting on their tops. Lift your upper body up off the ground, inhaling through your nose as you rise. Press your hips into the floor and curve your upper body backward, looking up. Hold for 10 seconds to 1 minute.

day. To do these exercises correctly, use a weight heavy enough that you feel fatigued by the 12th repetition. Switch back and forth between the two exercises for a total of four times for each exercise without resting. Make sure you warm up before you strength train, and do the three cooldown stretches in "Warmup and Cooldown." Use your daily exercise log to help you check off each set you perform. As the 12 repetitions get easier, move up to a heavier weight so that you continue to make rapid progress. Not all of the exercises require a dumbbell, so you can leave the "pounds" column blank for those exercises. As you progress through the program, you may want to add wrist or ankle weights to them. In that case, use the "pounds" column to record that weight. The log isn't helpful if you don't use it, so keep a pen handy!

Frequently Asked Questions

What if I stop seeing progress during the 8 Minutes in the Morning program?

If this happens to you, just focus on what you want immediately. Don't waste time focusing on the problem. Ask yourself if you are following the Eating Card System precisely and doing your 8 Minutes in the Morning workouts consistently. If so, then you may need to "jump-start" your success by doing two things. First, follow the Quick Start portion of the Eating Card for the next 7 days. At the same time, if you are not feeling fatigued by the 12th repetition of your morning strength-training exercises, start using heavier dumbbells.

3. Use the Eating Card System found starting on page 233. Photocopy the cards you need for the week, and always carry them with you to help you keep track of your portions (see page 70 to review how to use the Eating Cards). Be sure to read the food tip each day, which will help you Eat Fat to Get Fit. Use the journal space at the end of each day to write down your thoughts and breakthroughs while living this program. This book is meant to be interactive and cannot be finalized without your input. Writing your goals and thoughts will personalize your program. Keeping a journal will teach you more about you. When you add the information that is uniquely yours, this book will be the most important book you own.

I recommend that you start the program on a Monday. That will allow you to take every Sunday off from exercising (but keep using your Eating Cards), giving you an opportunity to rest, weigh in, and prepare for the next week. If you have completed all the tasks on the list below, then you're ready to get started on your first day of the program.

- Have your dumbbells, a chair, and a mat or towel ready for action.
- Photocopy the master Eating Cards from page 234.
- Have comfortable clothes on.
- Have your "before" photo taken and taped on page 23. If you have not yet taken it, do it today! This will serve as one of the best ways to accurately assess your progress.
- Have filled out the Success Contract on page 28; if you haven't finished it, do that now! This will help you stay focused and committed to your goal.

Let's go!

Week 1
Day 1

"When health is absent

Wisdom cannot reveal itself,

Art cannot become manifest,

Strength cannot be exerted,

Wealth is useless, and

Reason is powerless."

—Herophilies, 300 B.C.

Know What You Want

Have you ever known someone who was so passionate and emotional that nothing could stand in the way? Throughout history, people such as Thomas Edison, Henry Ford, the Wright brothers, Bill Gates, and Mother Teresa all had a passion so strong that no matter the obstacles, they made their dreams come true. What was their secret to staying so driven? How did they ignite their passion every day? They each had a very clear plan, a mental blueprint, that guided them successfully to their targets.

You need a similar passion to build your dream body. Having a mental blueprint is critical to your success. With a clear target, you have the most powerful advantage to making your dream body a reality. Imagine trying to build a house without a blueprint or traveling to a new place without a road map.

Start by designing your ultimate body. Grab a pen and write down what your new body will look like in "What Is My Specific Goal?" Will you have a defined face, sculpted arms, lean legs, a flat stomach? *Imagine the ideal you and describe what you see.* When you finish, start your 8 Minutes in the Morning workout.

What Is My Specific Goal?

_____

_____

_____

_____

_____

_____

_____

Do a quick warmup before starting. Do one set of 12 repetitions from exercise A, then immediately do one set of 12 reps from exercise B. Repeat the cycle for a total of four sets of each exercise, checking them off on your log as you go. Then do the three cooldown stretches.

Exercise Log

Exercise	lb	Set 1 (✓)	Set 2 (✓)	Set 3 (✓)	Set 4 (✓)
A					
B					

EXERCISE A: CHEST
Dumbbell Press

Lie on a mat on your back with your knees bent and your feet flat on the floor. You may place one or more pillows under your back and head for support. Holding a dumbbell in each hand, bring your elbows in line with your shoulders, making a right angle between your upper arm and your side. Exhale as you slowly extend your arms and press the dumbbells toward the ceiling. Keep your elbows slightly bent. Hold for 1 second. Inhale as you return to the starting point.

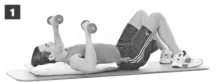

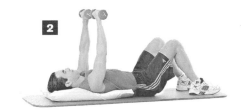

EXERCISE B: BACK
Two-Arm Row

Sit in a sturdy chair and grasp a dumbbell in each hand. You may put a pillow on your lap for support. Lean forward and extend your arms straight down, being sure to keep your elbows slightly bent. Exhale as you slowly bend your elbows and bring them toward the ceiling. Once the dumbbells reach the top of your thigh, hold for 1 second. Inhale as you slowly lower the dumbbells to the starting point.

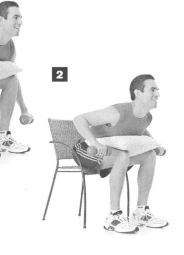

Dehydration can slow your metabolism by 3 percent. If you weigh 150 pounds, that amounts to 45 fewer calories burned each day. That's the amount in 1 tablespoon of pancake syrup. Even though that doesn't sound like a lot, think in the long term. That 45 calories a day can keep your body from burning 5 pounds of fat a year. It adds up!

Few people drink as much water as they should. If you feel thirsty, you are already dehydrated, so don't rely on your body to tell you when to drink. Instead, drink water on a regular basis. Keep a large water bottle at your desk and take generous sips frequently. Drink a tall glass of water before and after your 8 Minutes in the Morning workout, at your lunch break, and before dinner.

Today's Journal

_____

_____

_____

_____

_____

_____

_____

_____

_____

_____

_____

_____

_____

Week 1
Day 2

"The future depends on

what we do in the present."

—Mahatma Gandhi,
Indian nationalist leader

Get Dissatisfied Now

Remember the character Ebenezer Scrooge in Charles Dickens's *A Christmas Carol*? Scrooge was a selfish and mean old man who changed his behavior literally overnight, waking the next day ready for a better life after three ghosts visited him and pointed out his evil ways. When he looked at his life as an observer rather than as a participant, he felt so bad about his actions that he said, "Enough!"

Have you ever been so angry, sad, or disappointed at something you had been doing that you finally said, "Enough! I will no longer do this!" That is what you must do right now. Make dissatisfaction work for you. It is one of the most valuable motivational tools you can use to ignite that spark inside you.

What has being fat and unfit cost you in your career, your intimate relationships, your family relationships, and your personal happiness? Be honest with yourself. Dissatisfaction can provide you with the genesis of your success. Take a few minutes right now to capture your feelings about what inactivity and overeating have cost you. Pick up your pen and write them down in "What Pain Has Being Unfit Caused Me?"

What Pain Has Being Unfit Caused Me?

_____

_____

_____

_____

_____

_____

_____

_____

Do a quick warmup before starting. Do one set of 12 repetitions from exercise A, then immediately do one set of 12 reps from exercise B. Repeat the cycle for a total of four sets of each exercise, checking them off on your log as you go. Then do the three cooldown stretches.

Exercise Log

Exercise	lb	Set 1 (✓)	Set 2 (✓)	Set 3 (✓)	Set 4 (✓)
A					
B					

EXERCISE A:
SHOULDERS
Lateral Raise

Stand with your feet shoulder-width apart, your back straight, and your abs tight. Hold a dumbbell in each hand at your sides with your arms straight and your elbows slightly bent. Exhale as you slowly lift the dumbbells out to the side until they are slightly above shoulder level and your palms are facing the floor. Hold for 1 second. Inhale as you lower your arms to the starting point.

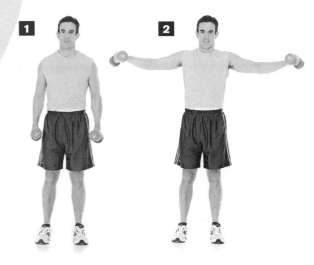

EXERCISE B:
ABDOMINALS
Crunch

Lie on a mat on your back with your knees bent and your feet flat on the floor. Make a fist with one hand and place it between your chin and collarbone. With your other hand, grasp your wrist. This will prevent you from leading with your head and straining your neck. Without moving your lower body, exhale and slowly curl your upper torso until your shoulder blades are off the ground. Hold for 1 second. Inhale as you slowly lower yourself to the starting position.

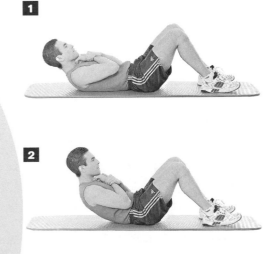

TODAY'S MOVES

WEEK 1 ▶ DAY 2

A lot of people overeat not because they are hungry but simply because the food is there. To help yourself stick to the portions that correspond to your calorie selection, dish the correct portions onto your plate and leave the rest of the food in the kitchen. Don't bring it to the table where you might be tempted to indulge in seconds.

Do the same with your snacks. Buy your "Treats and Cravings" items such as chips and sweets in small packs or individual servings so that you won't be tempted to down a family-size package while you watch TV or talk on the phone. And never *ever* eat ice cream straight from the container.

Today's Journal

_____

_____

_____

_____

_____

_____

_____

_____

_____

_____

_____

_____

Week 1
Day 3

"Obstacles don't have to stop you. If you run into a wall, don't turn around and give up. Figure out how to climb it, go through it, or work around it."

—Michael Jordan,
U.S. basketball player

Know What You Will Gain

For many years, Randy Leamer had unsuccessfully tried to lose weight. But then one day, he became *very* motivated. Within a year, he lost more than 103 pounds. How did he do it? Where did he find that motivation?

Randy had what I call a Passion Reason (PR). His 5-year-old daughter was in serious need of a kidney transplant, and Randy was the only match. But

My Power List
1. _____
PR: _____
PR: _____
2. _____
PR: _____
PR: _____
3. _____
PR: _____
PR: _____

he was so obese that doctors didn't want to perform the surgery; it was too risky. So without hesitation, Randy started eating properly and exercising daily. For the next 11 months, he never complained and never missed a workout. Once he lost the weight, he was able to donate his kidney and save his daughter's life. He has kept the weight off ever since.

You must find your own Passion Reasons by creating a Power List. Write down the three most important things in your life—your spouse, your family, financial freedom, your spirituality, and so on.

Then ask yourself what you will gain by losing weight. Your answer to that question will help you create Passion Reasons (two for each item on your list). If you put your spouse on your Power List, you might answer "more romance and better sex." If it's financial independence, you might write down "more energy to start home business." Review your Passion Reasons every day!

Do a quick warmup before starting. Do one set of 12 repetitions from exercise A, then immediately do one set of 12 reps from exercise B. Repeat the cycle for a total of four sets of each exercise, checking them off on your log as you go. Then do the three cooldown stretches.

Exercise Log

Exercise	lb	Set 1 (✓)	Set 2 (✓)	Set 3 (✓)	Set 4 (✓)
A					
B					

EXERCISE A: TRICEPS
Lying Kickback

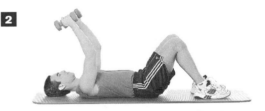

Lie on a mat on your back with a dumbbell in each hand by your ears and your elbows pointing up. Exhale as you slowly extend your arms and raise the dumbbells toward the ceiling. Straighten your arms but keep your elbows slightly bent. Hold for 1 second. Inhale as you lower the dumbbells to the starting point.

EXERCISE B: BICEPS
Standing Curl

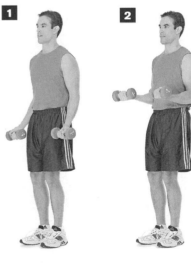

Stand with your feet shoulder-width apart and your arms extended by your sides. Hold a dumbbell in each hand, palms facing forward. Exhale as you simultaneously curl both arms to just past 90 degrees, bringing your palms toward your biceps. Keep your elbows close to your sides and concentrate on moving only from your elbow joints, not from your shoulders. Hold for 1 second. Inhale as you return to the starting point.

TODAY'S MOVES   WEEK 1 ▶ DAY 3

Even though fruit juice is loaded with vitamins and antioxidants that can improve your health, most types are also loaded with calories. One 10-ounce bottle can contain 150 calories. If you love juice and want its nutritional goodness but don't want the calories, dilute it. Fill your glass halfway with sparkling water and the rest of the way with your fruit juice. That will cut the calorie count in half without sacrificing the taste. You can also add sparkling water to wine, tomato juice, and even soda. Over time, you can wean yourself from caloric drinks altogether by increasing the amount of sparkling water. Eventually, you'll be drinking sparkling water with only a hint of juice or soda for taste.

Today's Journal

_____

_____

_____

_____

_____

_____

_____

_____

_____

_____

_____

_____

"When you always do your best, you take action. Doing your best is taking action because you love it, not because you're expecting a reward."

—Don Miguel Ruiz,
author of *The Four Agreements*

See It and Make It Real

Being able to vividly see your ideal body is a critical step in achieving that body. Think about any item in the physical world: a car, a computer, or a dress. It did not get here by accident. It's here because someone saw a very clear mental image of what they wanted to create before it existed.

That is what I want to you to experience right now. I want you to see the body that you will have in the future. Practicing visualization (see "Visualization Exercise") each morning will allow you to see and feel the new you that is emerging.

Visualization Exercise

1. Close your eyes; take a few deep, relaxing breaths through your nose; and see yourself through the lens of a camera. Look at yourself with the body you want to have. How is your posture? What are you wearing? If you are seeing a black-and-white picture of yourself, add color. Put a big smile on your face.

2. With your eyes still closed, see yourself through the lens of a video camera. This means that you can stretch, walk, dance, run, laugh, or interact with the environment you are in. See the body you want to have.

3. Jump into the body that you want. You can now see things through your own eyes. Look at the tone in your arms and legs; it is yours to enjoy.

Do a quick warmup before starting. Do one set of 12 repetitions from exercise A, then immediately do one set of 12 reps from exercise B. Repeat the cycle for a total of four sets of each exercise, checking them off on your log as you go. Then do the three cooldown stretches.

Exercise Log

Exercise	lb	Set 1 (✓)	Set 2 (✓)	Set 3 (✓)	Set 4 (✓)
A					
B					

EXERCISE A:
HAMSTRINGS
Hamstring Leg Lift

Lie on a mat with your palms flat on the floor and your heels on the seat of a sturdy chair. Exhale as you slowly contract the backs of your upper thighs to push your butt toward the ceiling. Hold for 1 second. Inhale as you slowly lower your butt to the starting point.

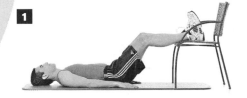
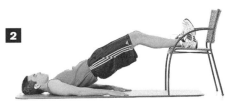

EXERCISE B:
QUADRICEPS
Squat

Stand with your feet slightly wider than shoulder-width apart and your arms at your sides. Keeping your back straight and your abs tight, exhale as you slowly squat down to about 90 degrees. Push your butt out as if you were sitting into a chair and don't let your knees extend forward past your toes. If you need to, you can rest your hands on your thighs. Hold for 1 second. Inhale as you slowly return to the starting position.

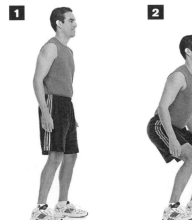
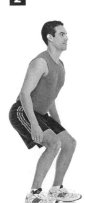

Olive oil is one of the more healthful oils to cook with, which is why I recommend it in my Eat Fat to Get Fit eating program. There are many varieties, and it can be overwhelming to choose which one you want to try. From regular to virgin to extra-virgin, the best one really depends on your taste buds and your budget.

Extra-virgin is the most expensive and highest-quality olive oil. To qualify as extra-virgin, the olives must have been handpicked at the optimum ripeness, giving the oil a rich flavor. When a bottle is labeled just "olive oil," it contains some imperfections, lacks some of the rich flavor of extra-virgin, and costs less. "Virgin" olive oil falls somewhere between extra-virgin and plain when it comes to taste and quality. "Light" olive oil is not light in calories, but light in taste and appearance. It's designed specifically for people who want to use olive oil but don't like its strong taste.

Today's Journal

_____

_____

_____

_____

_____

_____

_____

_____

_____

_____

_____

_____

_____

Week 1
Day 5

"Vision: the art of seeing things invisible."

—Jonathan Swift,
Irish poet and satirist

Create the Ultimate Environment

Do you remember the movie *Forrest Gump*? It is about a man who leads an extraordinary life even though he is "handicapped." Forrest is able to make all his dreams come true because of the way his mother taught him to see the world. She helped him master the ultimate environment: his internal one.

She explained things in a way that made Forrest ask what I call Result-Driven Questions (RDQs). Instead of asking himself, "Why am I disabled?" "What's wrong with my legs?" or "Why I am I slower than all the other kids?" he asks questions such as, "Why did God make me so special?" or "Why am I so lucky to have these magic shoes?" or "How do miracles happen everyday?"

By asking Result-Driven Questions, you are actually unable to focus on things that make you depressed or unmotivated. You have no option but to see things in a way that empowers you.

If you ask negatively driven questions such as "Why is it so difficult for me to lose weight?" or "Why can't I lose weight?" or "What's my problem?" your answers will reveal all of the reasons why you can't lose the weight and will make you feel worse. Using RDQs will give you the power to direct what you see and hear; they direct your emotions toward the results you want. You need to read and think about the RDQs each and every day.

Result-Driven Questions

Photocopy these RDQs and place them on your refrigerator, at your desk at work, or on your closet door so that you'll see them often.

1. What joy will I feel when I attain my ultimate body?
2. How incredible will my life become when I am leaner?
3. What extraordinary things will people say to me when I am leaner?
4. How will I see my body transform with the healthful choices I make?
5. What can I do today so that my weight-loss plans run smoothly?
6. How can I continue to create a weight-loss support network?

Do a quick warmup before starting. Do one set of 12 repetitions from exercise A, then immediately do one set of 12 reps from exercise B. Repeat the cycle for a total of four sets of each exercise, checking them off on your log as you go. Then do the three cooldown stretches.

Exercise Log

Exercise	lb	Set 1 (✓)	Set 2 (✓)	Set 3 (✓)	Set 4 (✓)
A					
B					

EXERCISE A:
CALVES

Standing Heel Raise

Stand with your feet shoulder-width apart. Hold a dumbbell in each hand at your sides with your arms extended but not locked. Keep your chest out, your shoulder blades rolled back and down, and your abs tight. Exhale as you slowly lift your heels and rise onto your tiptoes. Hold for 1 second. Inhale as you slowly lower yourself to the starting position.

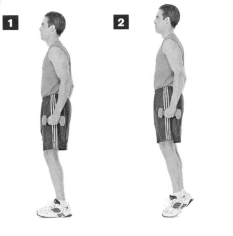

EXERCISE B:
BUTT

Kickup

Kneel on a mat on all fours with your knees hip-width apart, your hands slightly wider apart than your shoulders, and your fingers pointing forward. Keeping your head up, raise your left leg until your thigh is in line with your torso. Bend your knee and exhale as you slowly push your foot toward the ceiling. If this puts too much stress on your back, lower your head so that you are looking down at the mat. Once you've reached your maximum contraction, hold for 1 second. Inhale as you slowly lower your leg until it is once again in line with your torso. Do one set with your left leg, then switch sides.

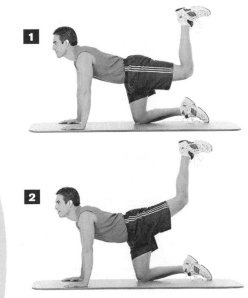

TODAY'S MOVES

WEEK 1 ▶ DAY 5

A lot of people tell me that they hardly eat anything, but still can't manage to lose weight. I ask them to think about all of those little calories that most people tend to think of as "freebies" or don't count as food actually eaten. For many, it's the food they taste as they cook. Those spoonfuls of soup, nibbles of cornbread, and snatches of cheese can add up to 100 extra calories a day. That could amount to an extra 10 pounds per year! Other overlooked calorie sources include free samples at the grocery store, goodies left on your desk by coworkers, and the rest of the food on your kid's plate. If you nibble here and there, don't forget to check off the right boxes on your Eating Cards!

Today's Journal

_____

_____

_____

_____

_____

_____

_____

_____

_____

_____

_____

Week 1 Day 6

"You cannot depend on your eyes
when your imagination is out of
focus."

—Mark Twain,
American writer and satirist

Create More Time for You

How great would it be if you could find an extra 3 to 4 hours each week? How could you use that time to accelerate your success? How much leaner could you get? How much sooner could you achieve your goal?

All of us have what I call a Loser Zone, where most of us spend too much time. You fall into the Loser Zone when you do something that produces no significant improvement in your life. The number one Loser Zone activity is watching television; the average American spends 30 hours a week watching it. Your Loser Zone time might also involve aimlessly chatting on the phone or surfing the Internet.

What are your Loser Zones, and how many hours per day do you spend per Loser Zone activity? If your number is greater than 6 to 8 hours, you have just found some time that could be better spent on creating your best body ever.

What Are My Loser Zones?

Loser Zone activity: _____ Hours per day: _____

Loser Zone activity: _____ Hours per day: _____

Loser Zone activity: _____ Hours per day: _____

Total time in Loser Zone _____ × **7 days** = _____

This is how much **MORE** time you have for yourself per week when you get out of your Loser Zone.

Do a quick warmup before starting. Do one set of 12 repetitions from exercise A, then immediately do one set of 12 reps from exercise B. Repeat the cycle for a total of four sets of each exercise, checking them off on your log as you go. Then do the three cool-down stretches.

Exercise Log

Exercise	lb	Set 1 (✓)	Set 2 (✓)	Set 3 (✓)	Set 4 (✓)
A					
B					

EXERCISE A: INNER THIGH

Inner-Thigh Leg Raise

Lie on a mat on your left side with your left elbow and forearm supporting your upper body and your left leg extended. Bend your right knee and place your right foot behind your left leg for balance. Keeping your left leg straight, exhale as you slowly lift your left foot as high as you can. Hold for 1 second. Inhale as you lower your foot to the starting position. Do one set with your left leg, then switch sides.

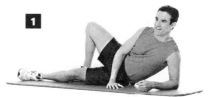

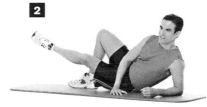

EXERCISE B: OUTER THIGH

Doggie

Kneel on a mat on all fours with your knees hip-width apart, your hands placed slightly wider than your shoulders, and your fingers pointing forward. Keep your back straight and your head up. Keeping your leg bent at a 90-degree angle, exhale as you raise your right leg out to the side (like a dog at a fire hydrant). Hold for 1 second. Inhale as you slowly lower your leg back to the starting point. Do one set with your right leg, then switch sides.

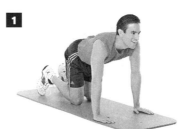

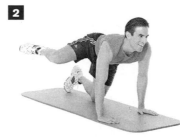

TODAY'S MOVES

WEEK 1 ▶ DAY 6

The next time you're in the mood for pizza, order it without cheese. Cheese accounts for most of the calories in the pizza, and it contains lots of unhealthy and fattening saturated fat. If you make your own pizza, use cheese substitutes made from soy, or use no cheese at all. I promise that you will eventually grow to prefer your pizza this way; I know I have. Now after I eat pizza, I feel healthy rather than bloated and sleepy. If you crave a hint of cheese, sprinkle a small amount of Parmesan cheese on top for the flavor without the bad fat and calories.

Today's Journal

_____

_____

_____

_____

_____

_____

_____

_____

_____

_____

_____

_____

_____

Week 1
Day 7

"You will never find time for anything. If you want time, you must make it."

—Charles Buxton,
American writer

Create a Power Collage

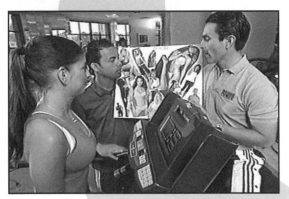

When you look through your old photo albums, do you feel the emotions captured in the photos? Imagine a special birthday, wedding, or graduation photo. Can you put yourself in that moment and feel it again? Photographs have a certain magical power for us; they can move us to feel a certain way almost instantly.

Have you ever seen someone in great shape and thought, "I want to look like that," then found yourself doing your next set of exercises with more excitement and motivation? You need to surround yourself with motivating images.

I want you to use your time on Sunday of each week to create a power collage. Flip through three or four magazines and select five or more photos of people who are healthy and fit that inspire you. Cut them out and paste them onto poster board. Put your power collage in a place where you will see it throughout the day and use these images to emotionally fuel your workouts.

This is your day off, so take some extra time for yourself. Go for a powerwalk, get some fresh air, and motivate yourself for next week.

8 Minute Marvel
Stephanie lost 32 pounds!

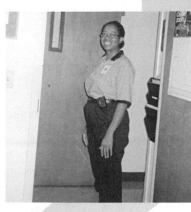

BEFORE

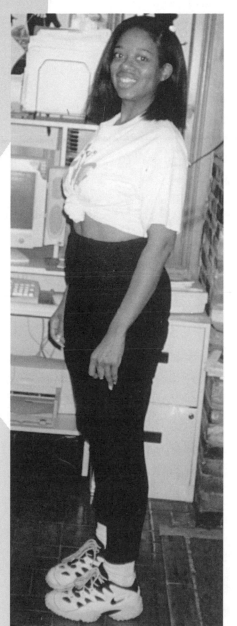

"A single mother of two, I've had an extremely difficult time losing weight in the past. After 2 years, I still didn't fit into my pre-pregnancy clothes. I spent months eating low-fat foods and doing 60 minutes of high-impact aerobics every day, but got nowhere. But everything changed when I started the 8 Minutes in the Morning program.

My body is now lean, and I have more energy than ever before. With the 8 Minutes in the Morning program guiding me, I always had the tools to accomplish my goals. This program has changed my life! My friends, family, and coworkers always compliment me on my appearance. New moms, this program works!"

—Stephanie Donald
Production Manager

L ike most people, I like to eat something sweet once in a while. But I don't like to check off all of those food boxes just for a piece of cake or a handful of cookies. So when I'm hankering for a sweet taste, especially just after a meal, I go to my freezer. Not for ice cream, but for frozen seedless grapes.

There's something about a frozen grape that makes it so much more delicious than the room-temperature version, and 10 medium grapes have only 15 calories. That means that you can eat 12 of them before you have to check off your fruit allotment for the day on your Eating Card. And grapes are loaded with healthful phytochemicals that fight off heart disease and cancer. That's a pretty good way to satisfy your cravings.

IMPORTANT: Week 1 Update

It's time to monitor your progress and record your 1st week's progress. This will keep you focused and accountable. Grab a pen and answer the following questions.

1. What is your current weight? Use a scale to weigh yourself and also write down your original weight. _____

2. What have you done well this week? What makes you proud of you? _____

3. What could you be doing better or improving? _____

_____

4. What is your game plan for week 2?_____

_____

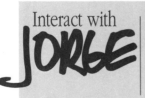
Interact with
JORGE

If you would like me to contact you about your progress, send me an e-mail with your answers to this week's update to weekone@jorgecruise.com. I will send you a special e-mail with bonus tips on how to make week 2 even more fun and effective.

Week 2
Day 8

"People only see what they are

prepared to see."

—Ralph Waldo Emerson,
American philosopher and poet

Create More Certainty Now

Feeling certain that you will attain your dream body is critical. A feeling of certainty is nothing more than a belief that you will do it. If you know that you will succeed, you will achieve it. How do you strengthen your belief that you will get a lean body? How do you create an unbreakable confidence that your goal will be achieved?

You need to create "positive references." Author Tony Robbins, my friend and mentor, explains the concept this way: Think of your belief as a tabletop and the legs of the table as the references that support the tabletop. For example, if you believe that you are smart (tabletop), you have references (legs) that support your belief. Maybe people have told you that you are smart, you have many smart friends, and you enjoy doing smart activities such as reading and attending seminars. Similarly, in order to believe that you will become lean, you need legs to support that belief.

Write down at least four references that support the belief that you will lose weight in "I Will Get Lean." For example, you might write: "I have so much to gain with my family," "I am good at completing tasks that are important to me," "I have the support of my family," and "I am a good role model for my kids." Review these references daily.

I Will Get Lean

My four references that support this belief:

1. _____

2. _____

3. _____

4. _____

Do a quick warmup before starting. Do one set of 12 repetitions from exercise A, then immediately do one set of 12 reps from exercise B. Repeat the cycle for a total of four sets of each exercise, checking them off on your log as you go. Then do the three cooldown stretches.

Exercise Log

Exercise	lb	Set 1 (✓)	Set 2 (✓)	Set 3 (✓)	Set 4 (✓)
A					
B					

EXERCISE A: CHEST

Knee Pushup

Kneel on a mat on all fours with your knees hip-width apart, your hands slightly wider than shoulder-width apart, and your fingers pointing forward. Bring your pelvis forward so that your body creates a straight line from your knees to your head. Inhale and lower your chest toward the floor until your elbows are even with your shoulders, keeping your back straight and your abs tight. Exhale and push back up to the starting position, keeping your elbows slightly bent.

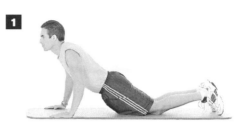

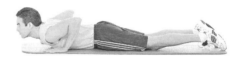

EXERCISE B: BACK

Bird Dog

Kneel on a mat on all fours with your knees hip-width apart, your hands slightly wider than shoulder-width apart, and your fingers pointing forward. Keeping your head up, exhale and simultaneously lift and extend your left arm and your right leg. Keep your back straight and abs tight throughout the move. When your arm and thigh are parallel to the floor, hold for a count of 3. Inhale as you lower them back to the starting position. Repeat with the opposite arm and leg. Continue to switch sides until you have completed one set on each side.

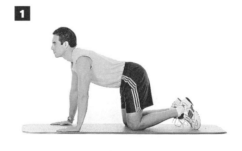

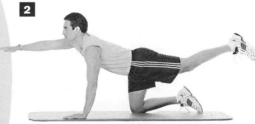

As part of the Eat Fat to Get Fit food plan, I recommend eating a lot of vegetables—no less than six servings a day and up to nine servings a day, depending on the calorie selection you are following. Some of my clients have told me that they have trouble fitting this many vegetables into their diets.

My answer to this is to keep cut-up veggies in your refrigerator at home and at work. Use them to satisfy your munchie cravings. Unlike snack foods such as potato chips and pretzels, you can eat as many crunchy veggies as you want. Just put a bag of baby carrots, sliced radishes, celery sticks, or cauliflower florets on your desk and nibble away. The best part is that you don't have to spend a lot of time preparing these veggies. Most grocery stores now sell prechopped vegetables so that you can eat them straight from the bag.

Today's Journal

_____

_____

_____

_____

_____

_____

_____

_____

_____

_____

_____

"You must do the thing you think you cannot do."

—Eleanor Roosevelt,
American humanitarian and diplomat

Create Your Power Label

I have a good friend who once worked at Disneyland at a concession stand. Although it wasn't the highest-paying job, she loved it more than any other job because everywhere else, she was just an employee. At the park, however, she was a *cast member*. She did not feel as though she was in the concession business, but rather that she was in the entertainment business. She smiled just thinking about her title.

> ## Power Labels
>
> | | |
> |---|---|
> | Sexy Mama | Strong Power Mom |
> | Adonis | Superwoman |
> | Hot Babe | Superman |
> | Athlete | |
>
> **Choose a Power Label (or make up your own) and write it below. Post it everywhere.**
>
> _____

This is what I call a Power Label. For you to achieve your ideal body, you must create a Power Label for yourself that gets you excited about exercising and eating well.

Think about it. Too many people unconsciously label themselves in ways that make them feel bad: over the hill, overeater, couch potato, sugarholic, meat-and-potatoes guy, or big as a house. The human brain is such a powerful instrument that you will eventually become whatever you label yourself. For example, if you really think that you have a "sweet tooth," you will always have problems with sweets. But the truth is that nobody really has a sweet tooth. It is just a saying that becomes real only when you take it on.

I want you to select a positive Power Label for yourself. Make up something that works for you. The secret is to live it everyday!

Do a quick warmup before starting. Do one set of 12 repetitions from exercise A, then immediately do one set of 12 reps from exercise B. Repeat the cycle for a total of four sets of each exercise, checking them off on your log as you go. Then do the three cooldown stretches.

Exercise Log

Exercise	lb	Set 1 (✓)	Set 2 (✓)	Set 3 (✓)	Set 4 (✓)
A					
B					

EXERCISE A: SHOULDERS
Overhead Press

Sit on the edge of a sturdy chair with your back straight and your abs tight. Hold a dumbbell in each hand with your hands just above ear level and your palms facing forward. Your upper arms should be parallel to the floor and your elbows bent at a 90-degree angle. Exhale as you slowly straighten your arms and press the dumbbells toward the ceiling, keeping your elbows slightly bent. Hold for 1 second. Inhale as you slowly return to the starting position.

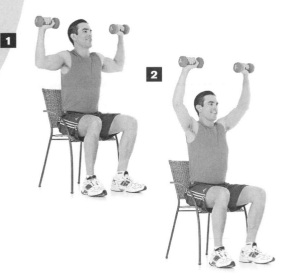

EXERCISE B: ABDOMINALS
Lower Pull

Sit on a mat on the floor with your legs slightly bent, your heels just above the floor, and your hands behind your butt for support. Exhale as you slowly raise your heels and bring your knees toward your torso. When your thighs and abdomen create a 90-degree angle, hold for 1 second. Inhale as you slowly return to the starting position.

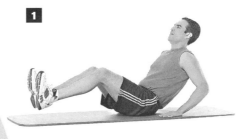

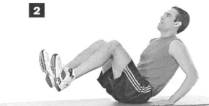

When people tell me that they don't like vegetables, I tell them that they probably haven't cooked them correctly. If you've ever eaten overcooked, mushy brussels sprouts, snap peas, or broccoli, you were probably left with a yucky feeling.

I challenge you to give vegetables another chance. This time, take care when you are preparing them. The best ways to cook vegetables are to grill, steam, or blanch them; or sauté them in an olive oil spray. Cook them only until they are warm; they should remain crunchy. Once they become soft, they will lose their taste and texture. Just like pasta, vegetables should always be al dente. You can also punch up the taste by adding lemon juice, garlic, or lime juice, none of which will add calories to your meal.

Today's Journal

_____

_____

_____

_____

_____

_____

_____

_____

_____

_____

_____

Week 2
Day 10

"People are just about as happy
as they make up their minds
to be."

—Abraham Lincoln,
16th U.S. president

Use Progress to Push Forward

Friends of mine have a baby boy named Matthew. I visit my friends once a year, and each time, I am amazed at how much bigger and smarter Matthew has become. But his parents don't notice and see the differences. It's not that they don't care or don't pay attention; it's just that they see him every day. When you are around someone or something every day, you tend to not see the small incremental changes.

It's the same with weight loss; people often lose their motivation because they think that they are not progressing. They think that their efforts are not paying off, which hinders their progress. One of the most essential things you can do to stay on track and motivated is to record your progress.

I want you to write down the 10 most important things you have learned while participating in the 8 Minutes in the Morning program. These are things that will help you stay fit for the rest of your life. They can be big things or small things. The secret is to notice that you have changed and then appreciate your progress. Use this list to remind yourself about the person you are now becoming.

10 Most Important Things I Have Learned

1. _____
2. _____
3. _____
4. _____
5. _____
6. _____
7. _____
8. _____
9. _____
10. _____

Do a quick warmup before starting. Do one set of 12 repetitions from exercise A, then immediately do one set of 12 reps from exercise B. Repeat the cycle for a total of four sets of each exercise, checking them off on your log as you go. Then do the three cooldown stretches.

Exercise Log

Exercise	lb	Set 1 (✓)	Set 2 (✓)	Set 3 (✓)	Set 4 (✓)
A					
B					

EXERCISE A: TRICEPS

Dip

Sit on a mat with your legs bent at a 90-degree angle and your hands about 1 foot behind your butt for support. Your fingers should face toward you, your arms should be slightly bent, and your butt should be slightly off the floor. Your butt should not touch the floor again until you are finished with the exercise. Exhale as you slowly extend your arms, keeping your elbows slightly bent. When your arms are extended, hold for 1 second. Inhale as you lower yourself back to the starting position.

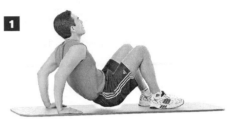

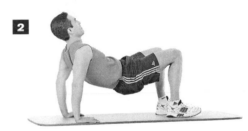

EXERCISE B: BICEPS

Hammer

Stand with your feet shoulder-width apart, your back straight, and your abs tight. Hold a dumbbell in each hand at your sides with your palms facing in. Keeping your palms in this position, exhale as you slowly curl your arms up just past 90 degrees. Hold for 1 second. Inhale as you lower your arms to the starting position.

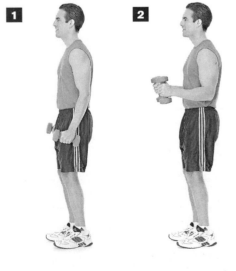

If you've never bought and cooked fish before, give it a try. Buy an easy "starter" fish such as salmon, swordfish, shark, or tuna. These all come in steak form, which is great for easy grilling, and are difficult to cook incorrectly.

When buying fish, look for cuts that are moist and firm with no dried-out edges. If it has skin, it should be shiny and metallic-looking. When you get the fish home, marinate it. For one of my favorite marinades, combine miso (a soy product) with some balsamic vinegar, olive oil, and a touch of low-sodium soy sauce in a resealable plastic bag, then add the fish. Let it marinate for 45 minutes before grilling or broiling.

Today's Journal

_____

_____

_____

_____

_____

_____

_____

_____

_____

_____

_____

_____

_____

Week 2
Day 11

"The door to freedom

is education."

—Oprah Winfrey,
American television personality
and actress

Jump-Start Your Motivation

I show clips of the movie *Cocoon* at many of my seminars to illustrate a point. The movie is about a group of senior citizens whose lives are turned upside down by space aliens. In the beginning of the movie, the seniors move like old people and feel unmotivated to live. But by the end, they move their bodies very differently—they climb trees, smile, kiss, ride bikes, jump, and even dance. When they begin to move differently, they feel motivated to do anything.

Moving your body differently can radically change how good you feel. Countless studies have proven that how you move your body influences your mood through your biochemistry. Hormone and oxygen levels all change with the kind of movements you make with your body. Try the exercise in "Jump-Start Your Day." It will have a dramatic impact on your motivation and focus.

Jump-Start Your Day

Do this exercise for at least 1 minute as often as possible throughout the day to enliven your senses. It's even better when you add some high-energy music.

1. Bring your hands together for a strong clap. With every breath, clap strongly. The palms of your hands have more nerve receptors than almost any other part of your body. Clapping your hands creates a neurological jolt that literally stimulates your brain.

2. Move into an energy posture. Stand up straight with your shoulders back and down and your chest out. This fully activates your diaphragm muscle (located under your lungs), which helps maximize your oxygen intake.

3. Jog in place. Breathe deeply as you jog in place. This further increases the rate of oxygen to your body by causing your heart to pump more blood.

Do a quick warmup before starting. Do one set of 12 repetitions from exercise A, then immediately do one set of 12 reps from exercise B. Repeat the cycle for a total of four sets of each exercise, checking them off on your log as you go. Then do the three cooldown stretches.

Exercise Log

Exercise	lb	Set 1 (✓)	Set 2 (✓)	Set 3 (✓)	Set 4 (✓)
A					
B					

EXERCISE A:
HAMSTRINGS
Leg Curl

Lie on a mat on your stomach with your arms crossed and your chin resting on your arms. Exhale as you slowly curl your legs until your calves are at a 90-degree angle with your thighs. Hold for 1 second. Inhale as you slowly lower your feet to the starting position. If you need additional resistance, wear ankle weights.

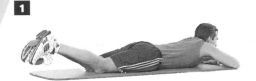

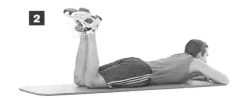

EXERCISE B:
QUADRICEPS
Lunge

Stand with your feet shoulder-width apart and your arms at your sides. Inhale as you step forward with your left leg until your thigh and calf form a 90-degree angle. Your left knee should not extend forward past your toes. Your right leg should also be bent to almost a 90-degree angle. Exhale as you push through your front leg to return to the starting position, then step forward with the opposite leg. Repeat 12 times with each leg.

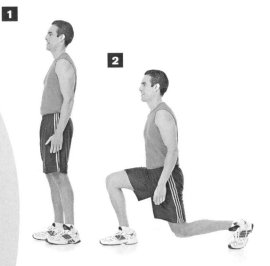

Some people ask me if they should switch from regular processed peanut butter to the natural variety, with the oil floating on top. It's a good move because the natural variety contains fewer bad trans fats than the more-processed types. If you're going to make a switch, I recommend trying almond butter instead, which can be found at health food stores and some grocery stores.

Most nuts are good for you, but study after study shows that almonds are among the best at fighting heart disease and cancer. They are among the highest in omega oils. On the other hand, some research shows that peanuts can be carcinogenic; fungus can be found growing in the shells, and they have fewer essential omega oils than almonds.

Today's Journal

_____

_____

_____

_____

_____

_____

_____

_____

_____

_____

_____

_____

_____

Week 2
Day 12

"Knowing is not enough;

We must Apply.

Willing is not enough;

We must Do."

—Johann Wolfgang von Goethe,
German poet, novelist, and playwright

The Power of Replacement

Do you have a bad habit that you wish you could eliminate? For me it was staying up too late. I knew that the best time for me to work out was in the morning, but at the same time, I kept going to bed at 1:00 to 2:00 A.M. Of course, I would not get up until 9:00 or 10:00 A.M. This was not my goal; I wanted to be up at 5:00 A.M., which meant that I needed to be in bed by 10:00 P.M.

To finally conquer this challenge, I had to replace the "fulfillment" I was getting from staying up late. I used to see staying up late as bonus time to work on whatever I had not finished that day. It was a magic time for me because I could get so much done. So I had to replace this bonus block of time with another block of time. I had to see going to bed late as a *waste* of my time. I now see my 5:00 A.M. wake-up time as more efficient (I can get in a full "East Coast" day and then a full "West Coast" day). It gets me more excited and thus motivates me to be asleep by 10:00.

Write down a bad habit that you want to stop. Then think about and write down what that habit has been costing you. What have you lost with this habit still in your life? Finally, come up with a replacement. It must be one that excites you as much as the old one. Write down how your life will get better with this new habit.

Replacing an Old Habit

Old habit: _____

What having this habit costs me: _____

Better habit: _____

What I will gain: _____

Do a quick warmup before starting. Do one set of 12 repetitions from exercise A, then immediately do one set of 12 reps from exercise B. Repeat the cycle for a total of four sets of each exercise, checking them off on your log as you go. Then do the three cooldown stretches.

Exercise Log

Exercise	lb	Set 1 (✓)	Set 2 (✓)	Set 3 (✓)	Set 4 (✓)
A					
B					

EXERCISE A: CALVES

Seated Raise

Sit in a sturdy chair with your feet flat on the floor and hold a dumbbell in place on top of each knee. Exhale as you slowly lift your heels, keeping your toes on the floor. You should feel this in your calves. Hold for 1 second. Inhale as you lower your heels to the starting position.

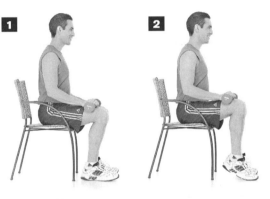

EXERCISE B: BUTT

Squeeze

Lie on a mat on your back with your palms flat on the mat, your feet shoulder-width apart, and your knees bent. Exhale as you press through your feet to lift your butt 3 to 6 inches off the floor. Push your pelvis up, flattening the natural S-curve in your lower back. Squeeze your butt for 1 second. Inhale as you slowly return to the starting position.

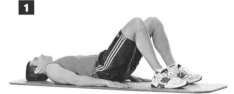

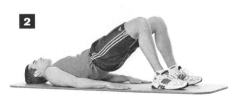

TODAY'S MOVES WEEK 2 ▼ DAY 12

Many of my clients (and many of you!) love butter. And most people don't want to give it up. There is room for all foods in the Eat Fat to Get Fit food plan, including butter, but I want you to try a simple switch for a few days. Fill a small plastic container with olive oil and put it in the refrigerator. The oil will harden, taking on the consistency of butter. Spread this on your toast instead of butter. It *will* taste different at first, but after a few days, your taste buds will grow used to it, and you'll actually come to prefer the olive oil.

Today's Journal

_____

_____

_____

_____

_____

_____

_____

_____

_____

_____

_____

_____

Week 2
Day 13

"Unless you change how you are,
you will always have what you've
got."

—Jim Rohn,
business philosopher

Create a Reward for Yourself

Today's Wake-Up Talk is simple and fun. Rewards are powerful motivators, so I want you to think of something you can give yourself at the end of your 28-Day Challenge. It must be something you love and at the same time must be something that supports your new lifestyle. It must also be consistent with the new person you are becoming.

My Reward

Here is a list of some simple rewards.

New outfit

A day at the beach

A day at a spa

Romantic dinner for two

Tickets to a show or concert

A new piece of sports equipment, such as a new bike or golf clubs

Pick something you really would love to give yourself and write it down. After you choose your reward, tell a friend or your spouse. If you can afford it, invite them as well. By getting them in on your reward, you get them to help you stay accountable and on track.

_____

Do a quick warmup before starting. Do one set of 12 repetitions from exercise A, then immediately do one set of 12 reps from exercise B. Repeat the cycle for a total of four sets of each exercise, checking them off on your log as you go. Then do the three cooldown stretches.

Exercise Log

Exercise	lb	Set 1 (✓)	Set 2 (✓)	Set 3 (✓)	Set 4 (✓)
A					
B					

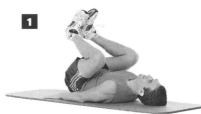

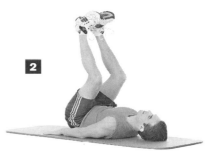

EXERCISE A:
INNER THIGH
Frog

Lie on a mat on your back with your palms flat on the mat by your sides. Pull your knees into your chest. Allow your feet to touch and your knees to splay to the sides, resembling a frog's leg position. Exhale as you raise your legs straight up, keeping the inner edges of your feet together. Stop before your legs are completely straight, making sure not to lock your knees. Hold for 1 second. Inhale as you return to the starting position.

EXERCISE B:
OUTER THIGH
Leg Raise

Lie on a mat on your left side. Support your upper body with your left elbow. Your legs should be extended and aligned with your upper body. Exhale as you slowly raise your upper leg. Hold for 1 second. Inhale as you slowly lower your leg to the starting position. Repeat 12 times with your left leg, then switch sides. For more resistance, wear ankle weights.

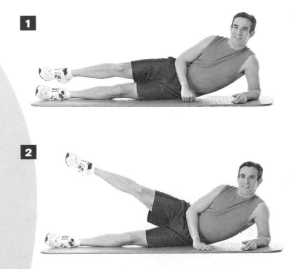

TODAY'S MOVES WEEK 2 ▶ DAY 13

The protein in dairy products, called casein, is an allergen that can cause asthma and sinus problems. I can vouch for that; as soon as I cut most of the dairy out of my diet, my headaches and asthma went away.

If you love to pour milk on your cereal and eat sandwiches with cheese, try switching to soy products. For every dairy product you can think of, there is a soy substitute. There are soy versions of milk, cheese, sour cream, butter, yogurt, and even ice cream. No, they don't all taste exactly like the real thing, but often, they taste better. And they are better for you. Sample different brands until you find ones that you enjoy.

Today's Journal

_____

_____

_____

_____

_____

_____

_____

_____

_____

_____

_____

Week 2
Day 14

"Hitch your wagon to a star."

—Ralph Waldo Emerson,
American philosopher and poet

Use the Power of Light

How do you feel when you are in the dark? Most people slow down and become tired. It's a biological fact: For thousands of years, the human race has gone to sleep when it's dark and has woken up when it's light.

You can use light to your advantage to stay focused and motivated throughout your day. Start using the power of light as soon as you wake up so that you feel your best during your 8 Minutes in the Morning workout. Adding more light to your day radically improves your mood and mental state, according to Dr. Bob Arnot, author of *The Biology of Success*.

Go through the checklist in "Bright Ideas" and start to incorporate as many as you can into your environment at home and at work. I guarantee that you will feel sharper and more motivated throughout the day. Then you'll continue to take the actions that will get you lean.

This is your day off, so take some extra time for yourself. Go for a power-walk, get some fresh air, and motivate yourself for next week.

Bright Ideas

• **Switch all of your home lighting to 100-watt bulbs.**

• **Go outside for a few minutes each day.**

• **Arrange your home to take advantage of open windows**

• **Leave your shades up at night so that the sunlight will wake you naturally in the morning.**

NOTE: If you would like to learn about light therapy, visit www.sunboxco.com (1-800-548-3968), and www.sltbr.org.

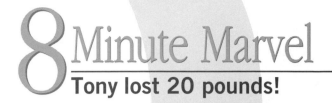

8 Minute Marvel

Tony lost 20 pounds!

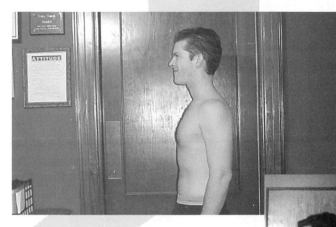

"I was having a hard time finding balance in my diet and exercise routine because of my seriously busy schedule. I had to find something that was simple and didn't take a lot of time. I found that with Jorge's 8 Minutes in the Morning program, just doing the exercises and eating right put me on the road to better health. It also gave me the right mindset to achieve all of the little successes that people in sales encounter on a daily basis."

—Tony Natoli
Salesman

BEFORE

f you like chocolate, you'll be happy to know that your body treats cocoa butter the same way it does olive oil. Chocolate does not raise blood cholesterol and can even improve your blood cholesterol profile. But there's a catch: Milk chocolate contains butterfat. Unlike other forms of chocolate, milk chocolate with butterfat can raise your blood cholesterol levels. It also contains very little cocoa compared to the more bitter dark chocolate. Cheaper chocolates often replace the cocoa butter with bad fats like palm oil or even partially hydrogenated oils. So if you're going to eat chocolate, buy dark chocolate made from cocoa butter and no fillers.

IMPORTANT: Week 2 Update

It's time to monitor your progress and record your 2nd week's progress. This will keep you focused and accountable. Grab a pen and answer the following questions.

1. What is your current weight? Use a scale to weigh yourself and also write down your original weight. _____

2. What have you done well this week? What makes you proud of you? _____
_____

3. What could you be doing better or improving? _____
_____

4. What is your game plan for week 3? _____
_____

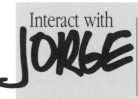
Interact with JORGE

If you would like to get more interactive, e-mail the answers for this week's update to weektwo@jorgecruise.com. I will send you a special e-mail with bonus tips on how to make week 3 even more fun and effective.

Week 3
Day 15

"Follow your bliss."

—Joseph Campbell,
author of *The Power of Myth*

The Power of Music

Think of a movie you really love. Every movie has a soundtrack that dramatically enhances it. Without music, a movie would not have the powerful emotion and energy that we all love. The same is true for getting a lean body. Music improves your workouts simply because humans are rhythmic souls; we naturally crave a beat to follow. Your heart has rhythm to it; your breathing pattern has rhythm to it. Once a beat starts, you want to start moving.

Music is magic and will make your 8 Minutes in the Morning workout much more enjoyable, guaranteed. The secret to using music is that it must have a continuous percussive beat so you naturally want to move. Latin music is my pick; that percussive beat is the heart and pulse of almost all Latin music. So, go out and buy yourself some new music. It can be Latin, but more important, it must be music you love.

Great Songs to Get You Moving

You can find all these songs on a CD I created called *Cruise Down . . . to a Leaner You!* It's filled with music hits from the '70s, '80s, '90s, and today that are recorded at 126 beats per minute (BPM), the perfect pace to complement your daily 8 Minutes in the Morning routine. It's also great for indoor and outdoor walking and any other workout routine that could use a boost of high energy. Listen to samples of them for free at www.jorgecruise.com/music.

1. Miami Sound Machine—"Oye"
2. Michael Jackson—"Wanna Be Startin' Somethin'"
3. Janet Jackson—"All For You"
4. Destiny's Child—"Independent Women"
5. Frankie Goes to Hollywood—"Relax"
6. The Gipsy Kings—"Bamboleo"
7. Merenbooty Girls—"Bien Pegaito"
8. Cheryl Lynn—"Got to Be Real"
9. Foxy—"Get Off"

Do a quick warmup before starting. Do one set of 12 repetitions from exercise A, then immediately do one set of 12 reps from exercise B. Repeat the cycle for a total of four sets of each exercise, checking them off on your log as you go. Then do the three cooldown stretches.

Exercise Log

Exercise	lb	Set 1 (✓)	Set 2 (✓)	Set 3 (✓)	Set 4 (✓)
A					
B					

EXERCISE A: CHEST

Fly

Lie on a mat on your back with your knees bent and your feet flat on the floor. With a dumbbell in each hand, extend your arms straight out from your body on the floor, palms facing up. Exhale as you slowly raise your arms straight up so that the dumbbells are almost touching each other above your chest. Your palms should be facing each other. Keep your elbows slightly bent. Hold for 1 second. Inhale as you slowly lower your arms to the starting position.

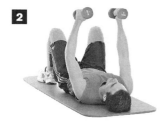

EXERCISE B: BACK

Standing Bent-Over Row

Stand with your feet shoulder-width apart. With a dumbbell in each hand, bend over so that your butt sticks out and your knees are bent. Extend your arms so that your hands are directly beneath your shoulders. Keeping your back straight, exhale as you slowly bring your elbows straight back, pulling the dumbbells toward your chest. Hold for 1 second. Inhale as you lower the dumbbells to the starting position.

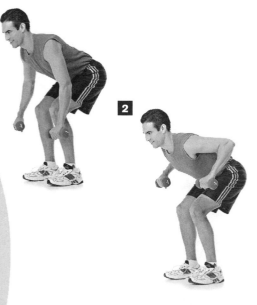

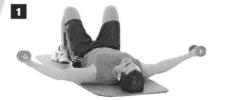

Is the rest of your family turning up their noses at your efforts to add more vegetables to meals? Then sneak them in. That's right: With a little creativity, you'll all be eating more vegetables without their noticing.

The secret to sneaking vegetables into family meals is to cut them into very small pieces and mix them into dishes that don't normally contain them. For example, you can mix chopped onions, peppers, carrots, and cabbage into meat loaf, or puree some vegetables and add them to pasta sauce. You can also add small vegetable chunks to your next casserole. The possibilities are endless.

Today's Journal

_____

_____

_____

_____

_____

_____

_____

_____

_____

_____

_____

Week 3
Day 16

"Nothing great was ever

achieved without enthusiasm."

—Ralph Waldo Emerson,
American philosopher and poet

Breathe Deep and Feel Great

What if you could use your everyday breathing as a powerful tool to boost your energy and motivation? Breath is the key to increasing your energy and focus because it is the only way that you can bring oxygen into your body. Without enough oxygen, you become lethargic, tired, and depressed. With increased oxygen levels, you not only increase your energy but also dramatically improve your mood. You simply feel better.

The secret to making your breathing more effective is learning how to "belly breathe." People in India have been doing this for hundreds of years. Belly breathing is the primary foundation for yoga and it is easy to learn. You will love how it makes you feel.

The key to belly breathing is using your diaphragm, a dome-shaped muscle located under your lungs. When you draw it outward (pushing your belly forward), it opens your lungs, drawing oxygen in. And when you push it inward by contracting your belly, you effectively move the used oxygen out of your lungs.

Try to use this type of breathing all day today, especially when you feel tired and lethargic.

Belly Breathing for Energy

1. Stand up straight with your shoulders pulled back and your chest pushed out.

2. Inhale through your nose for a count of 4 (make sure that your belly comes out), and hold for a count of 2.

3. Exhale through your mouth for a count of 5 (make sure that your belly contracts by coming inward).

4. Repeat for a total of 10 deep breaths. Do this whenever you feel worn out, especially when you think that you're too tired to exercise.

Do a quick warmup before starting. Do one set of 12 repetitions from exercise A, then immediately do one set of 12 reps from exercise B. Repeat the cycle for a total of four sets of each exercise, checking them off on your log as you go. Then do the three cooldown stretches.

Exercise Log

Exercise	lb	Set 1 (✓)	Set 2 (✓)	Set 3 (✓)	Set 4 (✓)
A					
B					

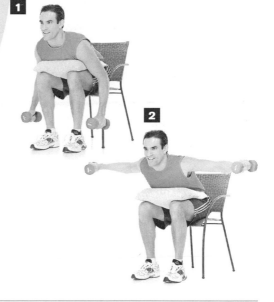

EXERCISE A:
SHOULDERS

Bent-Over Lateral Raise

Sit in a sturdy chair and grasp a dumbbell in each hand. You may put a pillow on your lap for support. Lean forward, making sure to keep your back straight. Your arms should be slightly bent at your sides. Exhale as you slowly raise the dumbbells to your sides, keeping your elbows slightly bent. Hold for 1 second. Inhale as you slowly return to the starting position.

EXERCISE B:
ABDOMINALS

Crunch

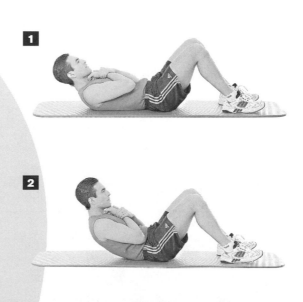

Lie on a mat on your back with your knees bent and your feet flat on the floor. Make a fist with one hand and place it between your chin and collarbone. With your other hand, grasp your wrist. This will prevent you from leading with your head and straining your neck. Without moving your lower body, exhale and slowly curl your upper torso until your shoulder blades are off the ground. Hold for 1 second. Inhale as you slowly lower yourself to the starting position.

As I mentioned earlier, saturated fat is one of the worst fats you can eat. One way to lower your intake of saturated fat is to switch from red meat such as beef to white meat such as chicken or turkey, which contains 33 to 80 percent less fat than beef. And of the fat in poultry, less of it is the saturated type than in beef.

But don't stop there. Most of the fat in chicken and turkey is found in and just underneath the skin. If you eat chicken with the skin, you double the amount of fat. Fortunately, even without its skin, chicken and turkey are still high in quality protein, B vitamins, iron, and zinc.

Today's Journal

_____

_____

_____

_____

_____

_____

_____

_____

_____

_____

_____

_____

Week 3
Day 17

"It is as hard to see one's self as to look backwards without turning around."

—Henry David Thoreau,
American writer

Be a Finisher

Having been through a challenging health crisis—and watching members of my family go through challenging health crises—I can tell you that becoming physically reborn is completely fulfilling. And nothing in life is as amazing as finishing something you set your heart on. It takes focus and dedication, yet nothing is as satisfying as changing your body and your life. But starting an important project such as getting fit and not seeing it through is burdening. It drains you.

My advice to you is to continue to take the higher road and be a finisher. The rewards are worth it. To increase your success, write down three difficult projects that you have finished. Examples include graduating from high school or college, landing your first job, getting married, or buying your first home. Get excited because *you are a finisher*. You *will* achieve your dream body.

Then write down the three worst things that will happen to you if you don't finish the program and get lean. Look 5 years from now, then 10 years from now. How bad will your life become? Use this dissatisfaction to push you to the finish.

3 Projects I Have Finished Successfully

1. _____
2. _____
3. _____

3 Worst Things That'll Happen if I Don't Get Lean

1. _____
2. _____
3. _____

Do a quick warmup before starting. Do one set of 12 repetitions from exercise A, then immediately do one set of 12 reps from exercise B. Repeat the cycle for a total of four sets of each exercise, checking them off on your log as you go. Then do the three cool-down stretches.

Exercise Log

Exercise	lb	Set 1 (✓)	Set 2 (✓)	Set 3 (✓)	Set 4 (✓)
A					
B					

EXERCISE A:
TRICEPS
Standing Kickback

Stand with your feet shoulder-width apart, your knees bent, and a dumbbell in each hand. Bend forward slightly, keeping your back straight and abs tight. Bend your arms at a 90-degree angle. Exhale as you slowly straighten your arms and press the dumbbells behind your butt, keeping your elbows slightly bent. Hold for 1 second. Inhale as you slowly return to the starting position.

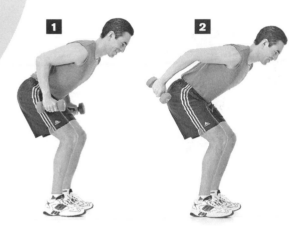

EXERCISE B:
BICEPS
One-Arm Curl

Sit in a sturdy chair and hold a dumbbell in your left hand. Bend forward and extend your left arm between your legs so that your elbow is braced against the inside of your left thigh. Exhale as you curl the dumbbell, bringing your palm toward your bicep. When you've curled your arm just beyond a 90-degree angle, hold for 1 second. Inhale as you lower the dumbbell to the starting position. Repeat 12 times with the same arm, then switch sides.

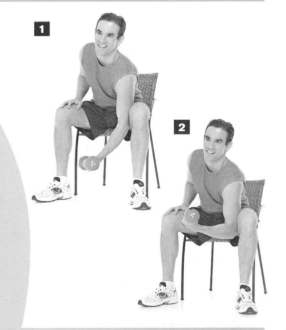

For many people, numerous unneeded calories come from what I call mindless eating. This happens any time you eat while doing something else such as driving, watching television, or surfing the Internet. Because your attention is elsewhere, you don't really taste your food or even register that you've eaten it. So you tend to eat much more than you normally would have.

If you want to chew on something while doing another task, I suggest sugarless chewing gum. Research shows that chewing gum can actually burn a handful of extra calories a day. But the best part is that it keeps your mouth busy. You can also try drinking lots of water or munching on low-calorie snacks such as celery sticks and cucumber slices.

Today's Journal

_____

_____

_____

_____

_____

_____

_____

_____

_____

_____

_____

_____

_____

Week 3
Day 18

"It is never too late to be what
you might have been."

—George Eliot,
English novelist

Focus on the Positive

In the process of coaching more than 3 million people online, I've discovered the most effective tricks to staying on track for the long term. It's all about knowing how to direct your focus. Your focus determines what you see and hear, which affects how you feel. How you feel determines your behavior.

> ## The Master Question
>
> **The more you ask yourself this question, the stronger your motivation will become. Use it every morning and throughout the day. I guarantee it will give you a powerful advantage in staying motivated long term!**
>
> **The Master Question:** *HOW GREAT WILL MY LIFE BECOME ONCE I AM FIT?*

This morning's Wake-Up Talk teaches you the most powerful technique you can use to immediately change your focus from negative to positive. By using this technique, you will instantly start to change how you feel. It's what I call the Master Question. (Recall the power of Result-Driven Questions from Week 1 Day 5.) You need to ask yourself the Master Question over and over again, almost like a mantra. Say it out loud or to yourself to focus your mind on success. This Master Question is simple and will immediately direct your focus on what you will gain. The more you use it, the stronger your motivation will become. Remember: If you ask, you shall receive.

Do a quick warmup before starting. Do one set of 12 repetitions from exercise A, then immediately do one set of 12 reps from exercise B. Repeat the cycle for a total of four sets of each exercise, checking them off on your log as you go. Then do the three cooldown stretches.

Exercise Log

Exercise	lb	Set 1 (✓)	Set 2 (✓)	Set 3 (✓)	Set 4 (✓)
A					
B					

EXERCISE A: HAMSTRINGS
One-Leg Curl

Kneel on a mat on all fours with your knees hip-width apart, your hands placed slightly wider than your shoulders, and your fingers pointing forward. With your head up, raise your left leg, keeping your leg extended. Once your foot is level with your butt, exhale as you slowly curl your foot to form a 90-degree angle with your butt. Hold for 1 second. Inhale as you lower your foot to the starting position. Repeat 12 times with the left leg, then switch sides.

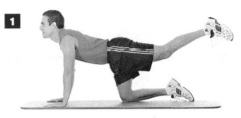

EXERCISE B: QUADRICEPS
Standing Raise

Stand with your feet shoulder-width apart and your arms at your sides. Shift your body weight to your right leg and raise your left foot until your left leg is bent at the knee at a 90-degree angle. (If you feel unbalanced, hold on to a sturdy chair.) Exhale as you slowly extend your left foot forward. Hold for 1 second. Inhale as you lower your foot to the starting position. Repeat 12 times with the left leg, then switch sides.

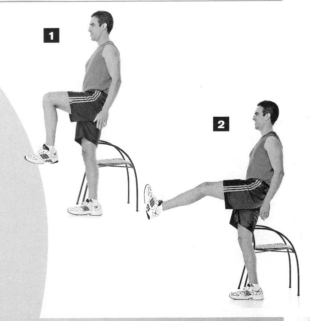

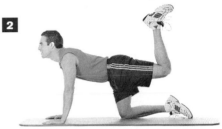

TODAY'S MOVES   WEEK 3 ▶ DAY 18

Tuna, chicken, shrimp, and crab are all great-tasting, low-saturated-fat choices of quality protein. But sometimes the way these foods are prepared can nearly destroy their healthful reputation. For instance, tuna, chicken, and seafood salads are all made with lots of mayonnaise, one of the worst condiments because it is high in cholesterol and saturated fat.

If you love tuna and chicken salad sandwiches, you do have an option. Make them by mixing the meat with soy mayonnaise, which is found in health food stores and some grocery stores. It contains none of the saturated fat of regular mayonnaise, but has all of the healthful benefits of soy.

Today's Journal

_____

_____

_____

_____

_____

_____

_____

_____

_____

_____

_____

Week 3
Day 19

"If you can dream it, you can do it."

—Walt Disney,
American filmmaker and animator

Feel Extraordinary with Serotonin

Today I want to share with you a simple trick that will help you change your mood for the better, jump-starting your motivation. The key is to change your brain's chemistry by naturally increasing the levels of a special neurotransmitter called serotonin. Research at UCLA has demonstrated that higher amounts of serotonin in our brains make us feel better, while lower amounts make us feel depressed and scattered.

The key to maximizing serotonin is not found in the drugstore or in Prozac or St.-John's-wort. It's in a smile.

The research shows that you can literally increase the amount of serotonin in your brain by changing your facial expression. For example, by smiling, you change the flow of blood to your brain and provide an internal environment ideal for producing serotonin. So if you want to immediately feel better, just smile.

Give Yourself a Reason to Smile

List 5 to 10 things that make you smile, from a heartwarming memory to a funny joke to sunshine on your face. Read your list whenever you need some help with your smile.

How has a simple smile changed your life?

1. _____
2. _____
3. _____
4. _____
5. _____

6. _____
7. _____
8. _____
9. _____
10. _____

Do a quick warmup before starting. Do one set of 12 repetitions from exercise A, then immediately do one set of 12 reps from exercise B. Repeat the cycle for a total of four sets of each exercise, checking them off on your log as you go. Then do the three cooldown stretches.

Exercise Log

Exercise	lb	Set 1 (✓)	Set 2 (✓)	Set 3 (✓)	Set 4 (✓)
A					
B					

EXERCISE A:
CALVES

Standing Heel Raise

Stand with your feet shoulder-width apart. Hold a dumbbell in each hand at your sides, with your arms extended but not locked. Keep your chest out, your shoulder blades rolled back and down, and your abs tight. Exhale as you slowly lift your heels, rising onto your tiptoes. Hold for 1 second. Inhale as you slowly lower yourself back to the starting position.

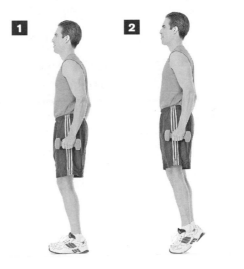

EXERCISE B:
BUTT

Leg Lift

Kneel on a mat on all fours with your knees hip-width apart, your hands placed slightly wider than your shoulders, and your fingers pointing forward. With your head up, raise your left leg and extend your knee until your leg is parallel to the floor. Exhale as you slowly bring your whole leg up as high as you can. Focus on moving only from your hip. If this puts too much stress on your back, lower your head so that you are looking down at the mat. Hold for 1 second. Inhale as you slowly return to the starting position. Repeat 12 times with the left leg, then switch sides.

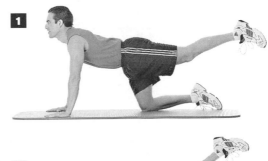

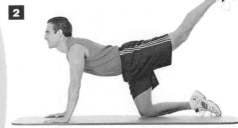

TODAY'S MOVES • WEEK 3 ▶ DAY 19

remember when the bagel craze was at its peak, with bagel-and-coffee shops everywhere I went. People couldn't seem to get enough of these treats. But what really amazes me is the reputation that bagels erroneously earned for being a healthful food.

While bagels are low in fat, they are not necessarily low in calories. The typical bagel contains a whopping 400 calories and accounts for 4 Complex Carbohydrate boxes on your Eating Cards. Worse, many toppings, such as cream cheese and butter, are high in unhealthy saturated fat.

That doesn't mean that you have to give up bagels completely, but I do recommend that you eat half of a medium-size bagel, which amounts to just 1 Complex Carbohydrate box on your Eating Cards.

Today's Journal

_____

_____

_____

_____

_____

_____

_____

_____

_____

_____

_____

_____

_____

_____

Week 3
Day 20

"The most wasted of all days
is one without laughter."

—e. e. cummings,
American poet

Find Metaphors That Get You Lean

Words and phrases can powerfully and instantly affect how you feel about things. You may remember from English class that a metaphor is a way to indirectly describe what something means. For example: "I am floating on air," "I am stuck between a rock and a hard place," and "I am at the end of my rope." You use a metaphor anytime you explain a concept by linking it to something else.

Here is the key: When you use a metaphor, you also are taking on the rules and preconceived notions that accompany that metaphor. In other words, the metaphors you use directly affect how you feel. If you use an empowering one, you will feel empowered. For example, instead of referring to exercise as a chore or work, think of it as a gift or as play. I've already come up with six power metaphors to help keep me (and you!) motivated to get lean.

My Power Metaphors

Use these power metaphors to stay motivated. If you think of others, e-mail the best ones to me at metaphors@jorgecruise.com.

My body is the most precious instrument I will ever own.

Food is fuel.

Exercise is a gift.

Life is a game.

My body is the temple for my soul.

Food is my medicine.

Do a quick warmup before starting. Do one set of 12 repetitions from exercise A, then immediately do one set of 12 reps from exercise B. Repeat the cycle for a total of four sets of each exercise, checking them off on your log as you go. Then do the three cool-down stretches.

Exercise Log

Exercise	lb	Set 1 (✓)	Set 2 (✓)	Set 3 (✓)	Set 4 (✓)
A					
B					

EXERCISE A:
INNER THIGH
Plié

Stand with your feet slightly wider than shoulder-width apart. Point your toes away from the center of your body, and point your heels inward. Grasp a dumbbell with both hands in front of your abdomen, at the midline of your body, with your elbows bent. Exhale as you squat down until your knees are bent almost at a 90-degree angle. If your knees extend forward past your toes, your feet are not far enough apart. Hold for 1 second. Inhale as you slowly rise to the starting position.

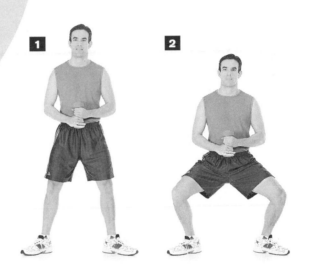

EXERCISE B:
OUTER THIGH
Pep Leader

Stand with your feet shoulder-width apart and your arms crossed over your chest. Exhale as you lift your right leg out to the side and extend your arms for balance. Hold for 1 second. Inhale as you slowly lower your leg to the starting position. Repeat 12 times with the right leg, then switch sides.

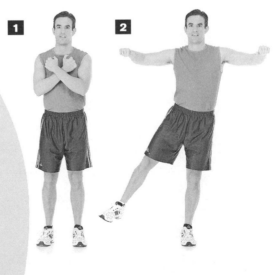

It's tough to watch your portions when you eat out. Restaurants routinely serve huge meals that can easily add up to 1,000 calories or more. And everything looks and tastes so good that it's hard to keep yourself from eating everything on your plate, even when you feel your belly bulging against your belt.

If you're with a friend, ask her to remind you to eat slowly and taste your food. It's a simple trick, but you'll actually eat less automatically because you'll be paying attention to what you're putting in your mouth. Also, as soon as your meal arrives, you can cut your portions in half and wrap up the extra food in a take-home container before you are tempted to eat it.

Check out other great tips in "Eating Fit at Restaurants" on page 72.

Today's Journal

_____

_____

_____

_____

_____

_____

_____

_____

_____

_____

_____

_____

Week 3 Day 21

"Shoot for the moon. Even if you miss, you'll land among the stars."

—Les Brown,
motivational author

You Are Who You Spend Time With

One of the most important secrets that will directly affect the quality of your health, fitness, and life is the idea that who you spend time with is who you become. It is probably the most valuable lesson I have learned in my life.

So when people ask me if they should join a gym or fitness club, I tell them that it is not necessary, but that it *is* critical to create some sort of support team. That could be a gym or fitness club, an online weight-loss chat group (such as the one at www.jorgecruise.com), a recreation or sports center (such as a YWCA), a healthy cooking class, or even a fitness book club. The key is to seek out people who are living life at the highest level, especially in regard to fitness and health. You want to surround yourself with people who are like-minded and interested in getting fitter. This is critical. It will help change your life!

This is your day off, so take some extra time for yourself. Go for a power-walk, get some fresh air, and motivate yourself for next week.

My Support Teams

Often, we don't achieve the best we are capable of because we put ourselves in an environment that never encourages us to be our best. Write down the names of people who support you, encourage you, and bring out your best, then make time to visit with these people on a regular basis. Also write down new places and environments that can help you meet more supportive people.

People who already support me:

_____
_____
_____
_____

New places/environments to support me:

_____
_____
_____
_____

8 Minute Marvel
Jill lost 15 pounds!

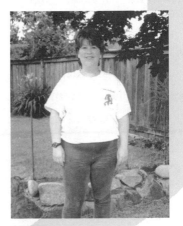

BEFORE

"When I first started 8 Minutes in the Morning, I weighed 150 pounds and felt unfit and fatigued. I had tried every diet out there and nothing had worked for me. But each week during 8 Minutes in the Morning, I lost an average of 2 pounds. As time went by, I could feel my posture improving. I was soon standing straighter and had more bounce in my walk. I feel terrific and I look forward to my workouts every morning; they help me start my day off on the right track."

—Jill Leonard
Telephone Service
Representative

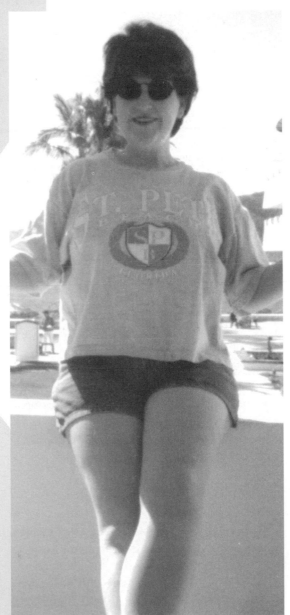

To start losing more weight, all you need to do is turn on your computer. You'll find a treasure of information on the Internet that can help you meet your goals. Although there are literally hundreds of helpful sites, I suggest you check out this one today:

www.vectrafitness.com. This website showcases my favorite strength-training home-gym systems, called the Vectra On-Line machines. You can adapt almost all your 8 minute exercises to any one of these excellent deluxe systems, with great comfort and safety. The models I like best are the 1600 or the 2850.

IMPORTANT: Week 3 Update

It's time to monitor your progress and record your 3rd week's progress. This will keep you focused and accountable. Grab a pen and answer the following questions.

1. What is your current weight? Use a scale to weigh yourself and also write down your original weight. _____

2. What have you done well this week? What makes you proud of you?____

_____

_____

3. What could you be doing better or improving?_____

4. What is your game plan for week 4?_____

_____

_____

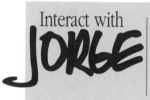

Interact with JORGE

If you would like to get more interactive, e-mail the answers for this week's update to weekthree@ jorgecruise.com. I will send you a special e-mail with bonus tips on how to make week 4 even more fun and effective—your best week yet!

Week 4
Day 22

"They always say time changes
things, but you actually have to
change them yourself."

—Andy Warhol,
American artist

Recommit to Your Success

The end of your 28-Day Challenge is almost here—just 7 more days to go! This is the day you must strengthen your emotional connection to what you are now doing—exercising and eating well—and what you will continue to do after your official 28-Day Challenge ends.

Recommitting is vital to your success today . . . and forever. If you are not fully connecting to what you will gain, you will lose your motivation. It's that simple. On the other hand, reminding yourself of your strong Passion Reasons will help you follow through automatically because you will *want to*, not because you have to.

Today, "raise the bar" another notch by rereading what you wrote on Week 1 Day 3 (see page 90). Then I want you to come up with seven more unique benefits that will create more Passion Reasons for continuing with the 8 Minutes in the Morning program.

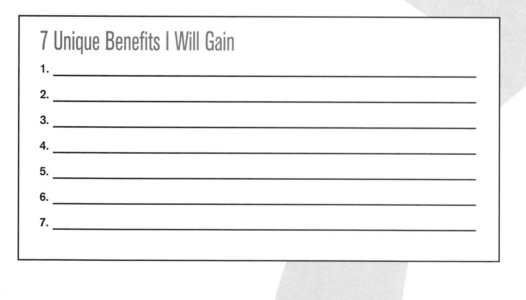

7 Unique Benefits I Will Gain

1. _____
2. _____
3. _____
4. _____
5. _____
6. _____
7. _____

Do a quick warmup before starting. Do one set of 12 repetitions from exercise A, then immediately do one set of 12 reps from exercise B. Repeat the cycle for a total of four sets of each exercise, checking them off on your log as you go. Then do the three cooldown stretches.

Exercise Log

Exercise	lb	Set 1 (✓)	Set 2 (✓)	Set 3 (✓)	Set 4 (✓)
A					
B					

EXERCISE A: CHEST

Pushup

On a mat on the floor, start with your arms extended but your elbows slightly bent. Your hands should be slightly wider apart than shoulder-width, and your fingers should be pointing forward. Your toes should be pointing down. Keeping your head up, inhale and slowly bend your elbows as you lower your chest toward the floor. Make sure to keep your back straight and abs tight throughout the move. Stop when your elbows are even with your shoulders. Exhale and slowly raise yourself back to the starting position. If you need to, you can do the easier Knee Pushup on page 111.

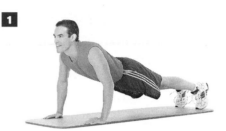

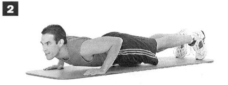

EXERCISE B: BACK

Superman

Lie on a mat with your belly on the floor, your legs straight, and your arms extended in front of you, like Superman flying through the air. Keeping your head up, exhale and simultaneously lift your arms and your legs about 4 inches off the ground. If this position puts too much stress on your back, lower your head so that you are looking down at the mat. Hold for 1 second. Inhale while slowly lowering yourself to the starting position.

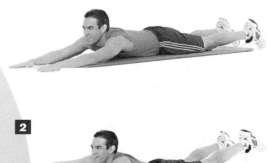

Bread is one of the most highly craved carbohydrates, but it doesn't have to be a guilty pleasure. If you eat whole grain bread, you'll be consuming slow-release carbohydrates that will keep your insulin levels stable. Be careful when shopping for bread because the packaging can be misleading. Just because bread is dark in color doesn't mean that it contains whole grains. Make sure the package says "whole grain" or "whole wheat." If it says just "wheat," it may still be refined. My favorite source of whole grain breads is Pacific Bakery (www.pacificbakery.com), which offers at least 10 great-tasting yeast-free flavors in the right portions for your Eating Cards.

Today's Journal

_____

_____

_____

_____

_____

_____

_____

_____

_____

_____

_____

Week 4
Day 23

"There are no shortcuts

to any place worth going."

—Source unknown

Walk Your Talk

Have you ever looked up to someone? Maybe that someone was a big brother, a big sister, or just a good friend—someone who served as a role model to you and who inspired you. A role model can be like a powerful treasure map that shows you the right path. A role model can serve as a blue-print for success and inspiration.

Who will be affected by the new you? Your spouse, kids, girlfriend, boyfriend, mother, father, best friend, sister, brother, or business associates? Make a list of all the people who will be touched by your new lifestyle. Then briefly write how their lives might change for the better by your being a positive and powerful role model. Get excited!

My Success Inspires Others

Who: _____ How: _____

Who: _____ How: _____

Who: _____ How: _____

Who: _____ How: _____

Who: _____ How: _____

Who: _____ How: _____

Who: _____ How: _____

Who: _____ How: _____

Do a quick warmup before starting. Do one set of 12 repetitions from exercise A, then immediately do one set of 12 reps from exercise B. Repeat the cycle for a total of four sets of each exercise, checking them off on your log as you go. Then do the three cooldown stretches.

Exercise Log

Exercise	lb	Set 1 (✓)	Set 2 (✓)	Set 3 (✓)	Set 4 (✓)
A					
B					

EXERCISE A:
SHOULDERS
Forward Raise

Stand with your feet shoulder-width apart. Hold a dumbbell in each hand at your sides. Exhale as you simultaneously raise both arms straight out in front of you. Move only your shoulder joints, keeping your back straight and your elbows slightly bent and stable without being locked. Keep your wrists firm throughout the move. When the dumbbells reach the level of your shoulders, hold for 1 second. Inhale as you lower your hands to the starting position.

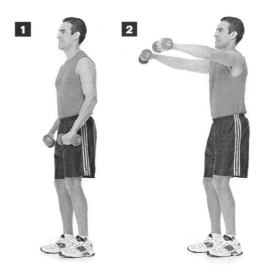

EXERCISE B:
ABDOMINALS
Lower Pull

Sit on a mat on the floor with your legs slightly bent, your heels just above the floor, and your hands behind your butt for support. Exhale as you slowly raise your heels and bring your knees toward your torso. When your thighs and abdomen create a 90-degree angle, hold for 1 second. Inhale as you slowly return to the starting position.

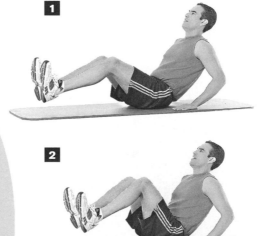

Very few people consume all the nutrients they need from food. Even if you eat a healthful diet that is rich in vegetables and whole grains, you may still be deficient in many important nutrients. That's because modern-day farming techniques have depleted some nutrients from the soil, making the foods we eat not as nutritious as they were in the past. To counteract these deficiencies, I suggest that you take a multivitamin every day. To find direct links to some of the best vitamins and supplements available, check out www.jorgecruise.com, or visit Dr. Andrew Weil's Web site at www.drweil.com for recommendations on different types of supplements.

Today's Journal

_____

_____

_____

_____

_____

_____

_____

_____

_____

_____

_____

_____

Week 4
Day 24

"If you find it in your heart to care for somebody else, you will have succeeded."

—Maya Angelou,
American writer and poet laureate

Move Forward by Saying Yes

You have only 4 days left before your 28-Day Challenge ends—I am so proud of you for coming this far! Do you realize that you are no longer the same person you were when you started this adventure? You have raised your standards and are becoming your very best. Today's challenge is to embrace the person you have become. Acknowledge all of the transformations that have happened up to this point. Capture all the big and small things that have changed. By doing this, you set yourself up to continue becoming the person you desire. By recognizing where you are now, you ensure that you will not block further success or revert to the way you were.

Write down all of the big and small things that have improved for you. How do you feel and look? How many inches are gone? How is your energy? What clothes fit again? What have people said to you? Pick up a pen and capture everything that is great right now.

What Is Great about Where I Am Right Now?

_____

_____

_____

_____

_____

_____

_____

Do a quick warmup before starting. Do one set of 12 repetitions from exercise A, then immediately do one set of 12 reps from exercise B. Repeat the cycle for a total of four sets of each exercise, checking them off on your log as you go. Then do the three cooldown stretches.

Exercise Log

Exercise	lb	Set 1 (✓)	Set 2 (✓)	Set 3 (✓)	Set 4 (✓)
A					
B					

EXERCISE A:
TRICEPS
Seated Overhead

Sit in a sturdy chair, grasp a dumbbell with both hands, and raise your arms over your head, keeping your elbows slightly bent. Inhale as you slowly bend your elbows and lower the dumbbell behind your head. Keep your elbows as close to your head as possible. When your forearms are parallel to the floor, hold for 1 second. Exhale as you raise the dumbbell to the starting position.

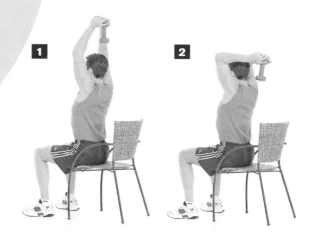

EXERCISE B:
BICEPS
Seated Curl

Sit on the edge of a sturdy chair and hold a dumbbell in each hand with your arms relaxed at your sides, palms facing out. Exhale as you slowly bend your elbows, curling the dumbbells up toward your shoulders. Keep your wrists straight throughout the move. When your arms are bent just beyond a 90-degree angle, hold for 1 second. Inhale as you lower the dumbbells to the starting position.

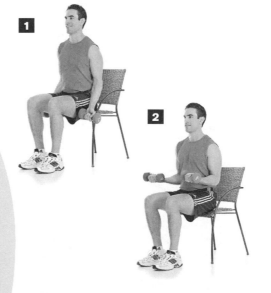

TODAY'S MOVES

WEEK 4 ▶ DAY 24

You can increase your chances of following your Eat Fat to Get Fit food plan if you consistently stock your kitchen with the right foods, including whole grains, fresh and frozen vegetables, olive oil, soy products, and beans. You can do that by doing a little planning before your shopping excursions.

Never leave the house without a shopping list. Keep your list current by updating it throughout the week as you run out of various foods. Before you leave for the supermarket, do a quick check to see if you need to buy staples such as beans, oils, or vegetables. And then eat a small snack. Research shows that people buy more foods that are unhealthful when they shop on empty stomachs. And try not to shop with your kids or friends; they can persuade you to buy food that will not support your goals.

Today's Journal

_____

_____

_____

_____

_____

_____

_____

_____

_____

_____

_____

_____

Week 4
Day 25

"Take heed: You do not find what you do not seek."

—English proverb

Resources: Web Sites

For the next 3 days, I will share resources for you to use to continue your success. Remember that the adventure you have been living for the past month is just the beginning. The best is yet to come!

Today I want to share some valuable Web sites with you. I have built my whole weight-loss career around the Internet, and I truly believe that it is one of the most powerful tools in today's world. Web sites allow us instant access to other people for support, the latest news on health and weight-loss trends, shopping, and great healthy-cooking recipes. Try to visit at least three of my favorite weight loss Web sites today. And enjoy!

The Best Weight Loss Web Sites

Check out this list of my favorite Web sites. Is there a site I missed that you love? E-mail it to websites@jorgecruise.com.

Eating
www.drweil.com
www.eatright.org
www.prevention.com
www.betternutrition.com

Exercise
www.acefitness.org
www.acsm.org
www.deniseaustin.com
www.ideafit.com
www.jacklalanne.com
www.kathysmith.com
www.goqlink.com
www.powerblock.com
www.stairmaster.com
www.vectrafitness.com

Motivation
www.ivillage.com
www.miguelruiz.com
www.oprah.com
www.oxygen.com
www.tonyrobbins.com
www.women.com
www.zukav.com

Favorite Gyms
www.clubone.com
www.crunch.com

Online Weight-loss Club
www.jorgecruise.com
(get a free 7 day pass online)

Do a quick warmup before starting. Do one set of 12 repetitions from exercise A, then immediately do one set of 12 reps from exercise B. Repeat the cycle for a total of four sets of each exercise, checking them off on your log as you go. Then do the three cooldown stretches.

Exercise Log

Exercise	lb	Set 1 (✓)	Set 2 (✓)	Set 3 (✓)	Set 4 (✓)
A					
B					

EXERCISE A:
HAMSTRINGS

Hamstring Leg Lift

Lie on a mat on your back with your palms flat on the mat and your heels on the seat of a sturdy chair. Exhale as you slowly contract the backs of your upper thighs to push your butt toward the ceiling. Hold for 1 second. Inhale as you slowly lower your butt to the starting point.

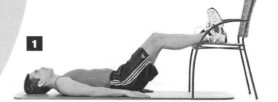

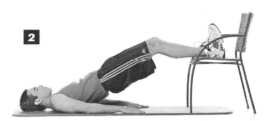

EXERCISE B:
QUADRICEPS

The Wall

Stand with your back against a wall and with your feet shoulder-width apart about 2 feet in front of the wall. Rest your hands on your thighs. Slowly slide down the wall, bending your knees until you are in a high seated position. Hold for 1 minute, making sure to breathe deeply while holding. *Do only one repetition for this exercise.*

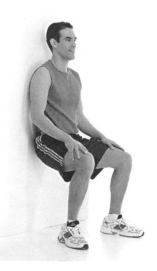

On my Eat Fat to Get Fit food plan, you're drinking eight or more glasses of water a day. Try to drink your water at room temperature because water that is too cold can put your body and organs into a state of mild shock. Some people end up with stomach cramps when they drink icy water, especially just after a workout or on a hot day. The contrast between their body temperatures and that of the water is just too great. Room-temperature water is also easier to drink in gulps, making you more likely to fit in those eight glasses.

Today's Journal

_____
_____
_____
_____
_____
_____
_____
_____
_____
_____
_____
_____
_____

Week 4
Day 26

"Project yourself into the probable future that will unfold with each choice that you are considering. See how you feel. Ask yourself, 'Is this what I really want?' and then decide."

—Gary Zukav,
author of *The Seat of the Soul*

Resources: Magazines

A magazine subscription is one of the best gifts you can give yourself and others because it is like having a good friend with great ideas and inspirational photos show up on your doorstep. It's a wonderful advantage to have an automatic source of inspiration and information enter your world consistently. It sets you up to win! When you least expect it or remember it, there it is in your mailbox. Today, check out some of the best magazines at the newsstand or in a bookstore. Flip through them. Eventually, I want you to subscribe to one of these magazines for monthly inspiration.

The Best Magazines

Do you have a favorite magazine that isn't on the list? E-mail your suggestion to magazines@jorgecruise.com.

Best Recipes
Dr. Andrew Weil's Self-Healing
    Newsletter
Eating Light
First for Women
Fitness
Men's Fitness
Men's Health
O, The Oprah Magazine
Organic Style
Prevention
Psychology Today
Quick Cooking
Self
Shape

Exclusive!
Read Jorge's monthly advice column in
First for Women

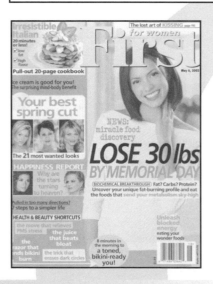

Do a quick warmup before starting. Do one set of 12 repetitions from exercise A, then immediately do one set of 12 reps from exercise B. Repeat the cycle for a total of four sets of each exercise, checking them off on your log as you go. Then do the three cooldown stretches.

Exercise Log

Exercise	lb	Set 1 (✓)	Set 2 (✓)	Set 3 (✓)	Set 4 (✓)
A					
B					

EXERCISE A: CALVES

Seated Raise

Sit in a sturdy chair with your feet flat on the floor and hold a dumbbell in place on top of each knee. Exhale as you slowly lift your heels, keeping your toes on the floor. You should feel this in your calves. Hold for 1 second. Inhale as you lower your heels to the starting position.

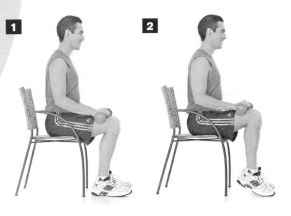

EXERCISE B: BUTT

Wide Squeeze

Stand with your feet slightly wider than shoulder-width apart, your arms at your sides, and your knees slightly bent. Inhale as you bend your knees to 90 degrees, making sure to squeeze your butt muscles. Hold for 1 second. Exhale as you slowly push through your butt back to the starting position.

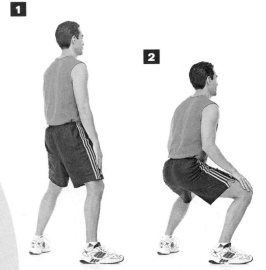

TODAY'S MOVES

WEEK 4 ▶ DAY 26

There's nothing like a cold or the flu to derail your best fitness intentions. Yes, you should rest while you're sick. But taking a few days off can get you out of your exercise habit, so try to stay as healthy as possible.

One way you can ward off a cold or the flu is by eating lots of garlic. It's a natural germ fighter and immunity booster, especially when you eat it raw. Try mincing a few cloves, placing them on a spoon, and swallowing them. Follow it with a sip of water. Mincing the garlic means that you don't have to chew it in your mouth and get that garlicky smell on your breath.

Today's Journal

_____

_____

_____

_____

_____

_____

_____

_____

_____

_____

_____

_____

Week 4
Day 27

"One can never consent to creep when one feels an impulse to soar."

—Helen Keller,
American writer
and social reformer

Resources: Reference Books

Books are great resources and with all the wonderful information, inspiration, and guidance you can find inside, they are sometimes like a best friend. Books have the power to change your life, as they are often the product of many years of study and experience from experts passionate about their messages.

I have many favorite books on my bookshelf. I recommend that, like me, you add as many as possible to your weight-loss library.

How essential is a good book? I keep a quote in my office from Erasmus, one of the greatest scholars of all time, who lived during the Renaissance: "When I get a little money, I buy books; and if any is left, I buy food and clothes."

The Best Weight Loss Reference Books

To order any of these books, visit www.jorgecruise.com/shop.

American Heart Association Quick-and-Easy Cookbook

As a Man Thinketh by James Allen

Awaken the Giant Within by Anthony Robbins

Flax for Life by Jade Beutler

Eat Fat, Lose Weight by Ann Louise Gittleman, M.S., C.S.N.

Eating Well for Optimum Health by Andrew Weil, M.D.

Everyday Cooking with Dr. Dean Ornish

100 Ways to Motivate Yourself by Steve Chandler

Powerfully Fit by Brian Chichester, Jack Croft, and the editors of *Men's Health Books*

Revitalize Your Life by Jack LaLanne

Strong Women Stay Slim by Miriam E. Nelson

The Taste for Living Cookbook by Beth Ginsberg and Mike Milken

Think and Grow Rich by Napoleon Hill

Weight Training for Dummies by Liz Neporent and Suzanne Schlosberg

Sleep Disorders by Herbert Ross

Workouts for Dummies by Tamilee Webb

Do a quick warmup before starting. Do one set of 12 repetitions from exercise A, then immediately do one set of 12 reps from exercise B. Repeat the cycle for a total of four sets of each exercise, checking them off on your log as you go. Then do the three cooldown stretches.

Exercise Log

Exercise	lb	Set 1 (✓)	Set 2 (✓)	Set 3 (✓)	Set 4 (✓)
A					
B					

EXERCISE A: INNER THIGH

Inner-Thigh Leg Raise

Lie on a mat on your left side with your left elbow and forearm supporting your upper body and your left leg extended. Bend your right knee and place your right foot behind your left leg for balance. Keeping your left leg straight, exhale as you slowly lift your left foot as high as you can. Hold for 1 second. Inhale as you lower your foot to the starting position. Do one set with your left leg, then switch sides.

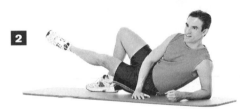

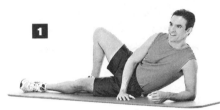

EXERCISE B: OUTER THIGH

Leg Raise

Lie on a mat on your left side. Support your upper body with your left elbow. Your legs should be extended and aligned with your upper body. Exhale as you slowly raise your upper leg. Hold for 1 second. Inhale as you slowly lower your leg to the starting position. Repeat 12 times with your left leg, then switch sides. For more resistance, wear ankle weights.

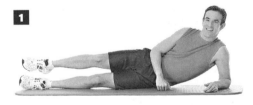

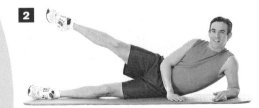

In keeping with today's "book" theme, I want to recommend *Diet for a New America* by John Robbins. After I read this book, I never looked at food the same way again. It will help you in your journey to Eat Fat to Get Fit, and I promise that it will give you a powerful advantage in your long-term weight loss.

Andrew Weil, M.D., highly regarded by me and millions of others, has stated that: "*Diet for a New America* should be read by everyone interested in healthy living. It is a well-researched, well-documented, and eye-opening account of the myths and truths about meat, milk, fat, and protein. I will recommend this book to patients, friends, and relatives."

Today's Journal

_____

_____

_____

_____

_____

_____

_____

_____

_____

_____

_____

_____

_____

Week 4
Day 28

"Nothing splendid has ever been achieved except by those who believed that something inside of them was superior to circumstance."

—Bruce Barton,
American advertising executive,
writer, and congressman

Celebrate!

You're finished, right? Well, not exactly.

You have been living a new lifestyle for 28 days. You now have a "lean machine" in place or are well on your way. But you must continue to move forward. By raising your standards, you are a new person. What once felt good will no longer feel the same.

Imagine that you never learned to walk and can only crawl. It would cause back problems and hurt your knees. You wake up every morning with a sore back and a feeling of fatigue. Now imagine that you have finally learned to walk. The pain and discomfort disappear. Why in the world would you go back to crawling on your knees? That's exactly how you must think.

Now that you have crossed the first 28-day finish line, celebrate and continue to move forward. Depending on how much more fat you need to burn, follow the 28-Day Challenge for another cycle. Each time you do, you will become healthier and fitter and feel better and better, guaranteed!

Grab a pen and write down exactly what you are going to do to commit yourself to living this new lifestyle.

This is your day off, so take some extra time for yourself. Go for a power-walk, get some fresh air, and keep motivating yourself.

What Will I Do to Continue?

E-mail your success story and photo to photo@jorgecruise.com. I look forward to hearing from you.

_____

_____

_____

_____

_____

_____

_____

_____

8 Minute Marvel
Lisa lost 20 pounds!

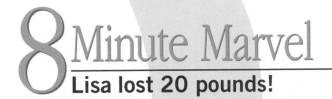

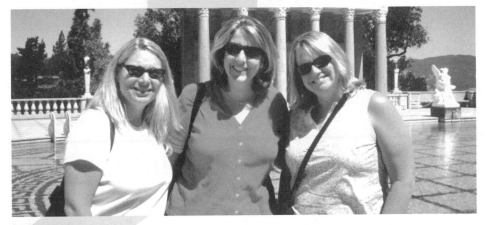

BEFORE (center)

"8 Minutes in the Morning is so easy to follow. I was even able to go on vacation for a week and still lose 1 pound, which has never happened to me before. This program has changed my life in more ways than one. I love the personal development. I am not only becoming thinner but also getting my self-esteem back. And the Eat Fat to Get Fit food plan is now a way of life for me. I used to love cheese, but now I don't even crave it. I have tons of energy and am very excited at my progress."

—Lisa DelVaglio
Sales Representative

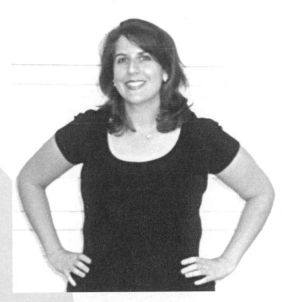

I'm not a big fan of salt—and neither are most doctors. Besides being connected with high blood pressure, salt also makes you retain water. So when you gain several pounds, it may well be from water, not fat.

Instead of seasoning your food with salt, try Spice Hunter's Zip Seasoning (www.spicehunter.com). It is a fabulous mixture of seasonings without all of the salt. You can also try an array of fresh herbs such as cilantro, oregano, basil, and more. Remember that cooking and eating are an *adventure*. Expand your tastes beyond salt and discover a whole new world of eating.

IMPORTANT: Week 4 Update

Congratulations! You did it! Now it's time to monitor your progress and record your 4th week's progress. This will keep you focused and accountable. Grab a pen and answer the following questions.

1. What is your current weight? Use a scale to weigh yourself, and also write down your original weight. _____

2. What have you done well this week? What makes you proud of you?_____
_____

3. What could you be doing better or improving?_____
_____

4. What is your game plan for week 5 and beyond?_____
_____

When you're done, have your "after" photo taken, then tape it to page 23 next to your "before" photo.

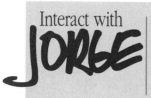
Interact with JORGE

If you would like to get more interactive, e-mail the answers for this week's update to weekfour@jorgecruise.com. I will send you a special e-mail with bonus tips on how to maintain and even further your success. Include your story, how much weight you have lost, how your life has changed, and what you are most excited and proud about.

CHAPTER 8

Your New Life
How to Maintain Your Success or Lose More Weight

You have just completed my 8 Minutes in the Morning weight-loss program. Great job, and congratulations on your success!

In my introductory letter, I told you that you would get hooked on this way of living. Remember how I compared your old lifestyle to crawling and your new lifestyle to walking? Now that you can walk, why would you go back to crawling? You've invested your energy and effort in making better choices that have helped you lose weight. You made choices that will keep you feeling and looking great forever. Keep up the great work!

So what do you do now? Whether you've arrived at your weight-loss goal or not, sticking with the program is the number one way to look and feel your best. If you still have weight to lose, simply restart the 4-week transformation cycle. Each time you go through this cycle, you'll get better and better results and that will ensure your long-term success.

But before you move on, I want you to savor your current success. Read back over your journal entries from the past 28 days. Relish how much you've changed and how far you have come. You have grown fit from the inside out. Treat yourself to the reward you wrote down on Week 2 Day 13 (see page 130). Now's the time to take that mini-vacation, buy a new outfit, or spend a day at the spa . . . you've earned it!

Keep the Weight Off

To continue the success of my 8 Minutes in the Morning program, follow these simple new rules:

1. If you want to keep the weight off or lose even more, you have to keep doing your 8 Minutes in the Morning workouts. Repeat the same exercise routine as you did for weeks 1 through 4, but *increase the amount of weight you are lifting.* This is critical! Remember that muscle gets stronger only if you push it beyond what is comfortable. And the more lean tissue you have, the higher your metabolism will be.

2. As you lose weight, switch to the calorie selec-

Frequently Asked Questions

When I do the leg lifts in your program, I don't feel like I'm working hard anymore. Is something wrong?

You've become stronger and your body weight is no longer heavy enough. Congratulations! To make these exercises more effective now, invest in some ankle weights with Velcro straps. I like the kind that comes with removable weights so you can continue to add weight as your body grows stronger.

tion that is appropriate for your new weight. When my clients achieve their ideal weight, I recommend that they switch to 1,800 or even 2,000 calories a day. This can vary, so do what feels healthiest to you. The Eating Card System will keep you honest, so use it.

Frequently Asked Questions

What do you think of alternative methods of exercise such as yoga and tai chi?

While they are not the most effective types of exercises for weight loss, these disciplines are excellent for variety and stress reduction. They will help focus your mind and spirit on inner tranquillity and peace.

3. Get on the scale to monitor your weight loss every Sunday. If you start regaining weight, jump to the Quick Start selection and follow it diligently to get back on track.

4. No matter what happens, never skip meals. Eat at least 3 meals a day, and always have fat with each meal. If you miss a meal, you are more likely to overeat at night. If you get hungry, snack on the unlimited vegetables (see page 215).

5. Review Your Wake-Up Talks. Your motivation needs to be exercised daily, too.

6. Remember that setbacks are only challenges in disguise. If you eat more than you should or you miss a day of exercise, just get back on track and focus on what you want. It's up to you, and you will do it!

Share Your Success: The Only Way to Enjoy Weight Loss

Probably the most valuable lesson I have learned from my 3 million weight-loss clients is that the way to truly enjoy weight loss and maintain your success is to share it with someone else. Giving someone else what you have discovered is one of the greatest joys in life. It's a privilege (and addictive!) to help others take charge of their lives and happiness.

My clients who lost weight and then helped someone else do the same are just as motivated months and years later as they were on Day 1. When you share your success, everyone wins.

In that spirit, I'd like to share the success story from one of my first clients, Joe Newsome. Joe lost 40 pounds with 8 Minutes in the Morning and then went on to help transform his family, friends, and coworkers. Here is his inspiring story:

"I've witnessed an incredible change in my life, a change that is so wonderful and is available to anyone who wants to become lean, healthy, and happy about themselves.

"I'm 5 feet, 7 inches tall, and before I discovered Jorge's 8 Minutes in the Morning program, I weighed

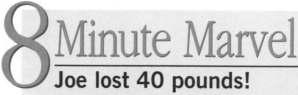

8 Minute Marvel
Joe lost 40 pounds!

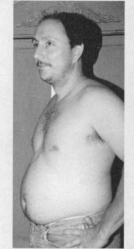

BEFORE

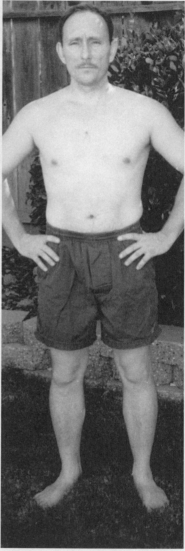

"I feel like I have turned the clock back. Now I do yard work shirtless and it feels great!"

202 pounds. I would trudge up the stairs to my house and feel winded. I hurt whenever I tried to run and play with my sons. I lacked the energy to get out of bed in the morning.

"A family history of heart disease scared me, and I finally decided that I would try to lose the weight, so I began my search for help on the Internet. I came across Jorge's Web site and liked what I saw. His program didn't include pills or chemicals. Instead, it focused on building muscle and eating the right kinds of foods *and fats*. All of the knowledge I needed to lose the weight was packed into one book and laid out for me on a daily basis.

"I started the program and saw results within the 1st week: I began sleeping better, my energy increased, my weight dropped, and I felt better about myself. The benefits just kept coming. My body began to start shaping up, the swelling in my feet disappeared, the pain in my joints began to subside, and I even stopped snoring. Best of all, I felt as if I had moved from my mid-thirties back into my twenties!

"My friends, family, and coworkers soon began asking me about what I was doing. Answering questions about 8 Minutes in the Morning soon became the focus of most of my conversations. The interest grew so large that I decided to form an 8 Minutes in the Morning team.

"I created a sign-up sheet, and 22 names later, we were ready to kick off our 28 days together. It was awesome as the support and inspiration continued to grow. Each pound lost was everyone's gain. Recipes, ideas, and tips were passed around through e-mail, and everybody inspired each other. We were one proud team!

"Sharing this program was an incredible blessing. I was attempting to pay back my friends and coworkers for all of the inspiration that they had given me while I was losing weight. But the benefits they achieved left me feeling so great and helped me grow even more with the program. It is one of the best feelings to share such a great change. Sharing in people's health and giving them a wonderful opportunity for a new, healthy lifestyle is the ultimate gift."

My Dream

In the Emotional Advantage chapter, I shared with you the power of having a specific goal. Well, it is my goal and greatest hope to be able to reach as many new people as I have already coached online. I want to change the lives of at least another 3 million people with this book. Remember that every 5 minutes, three people die in the United States due to problems related to obesity. And I can only do this with your support and success. By working together as a team, we can do this, and we will succeed—one person at a time!

What can you do right now to help make a big difference? Log on to www.jorgecruise.com/share and send a quick, but life-changing e-mail to all your friends about 8 Minutes in the Morning.

But regardless, please make sure to keep in touch with me directly at coach@jorgecruise.com and visit me at my Web site, jorgecruise.com, too. Send me your story and your "before" and "after" photos. Tell your friends and family about your success with the 8 Minutes in the Morning program, and before you know it, a worldwide revolution will be under way.

Above all, thanks for allowing me to be your coach on your amazing weight-loss adventure. God bless, and I wish you the best. I know you will do it!

Powerwalking

Exercising Your Heart

Though strength training is the smarter way to lose weight, you need to do some form of aerobic exercise to truly condition your heart and lungs. And compared to all other forms of aerobic exercise, walking is the most convenient way to get your heart rate pumping. That's why walking goes hand in hand with the core 8 Minutes in the Morning program.

My powerwalking plan will help you tap into "quick bonus" calories. Each time you walk for at least 20 minutes, you'll burn an average of 150 to 200 additional calories. If you walk 6 times per week at lunch or as an evening break, that could add up to 1,200 weekly calories, which adds up to an additional ½ pound of fat per week, or *2 more pounds of fat per month*. The bottom line is that adding powerwalking to your program will help you meet your weight-loss goals even faster.

So here is what I recommend: Always do the strength training in the morning because it is the most effective weight-loss solution, and fit in aerobic exercise when you have more time, want to burn more calories, and just as important, want to keep your heart and lungs strong.

Too often people who have a significant amount of weight to lose start aerobic exercise without first getting strong. Extra fat coupled with weak muscles makes aerobic ex-

Work Powerwalking into Your Day

Walking makes for a great break from your workday. Go for a walk on your lunch break to burn off stress, or do it after work to settle into the evening. To encourage yourself, and to get the most out of your powerwalking experience, try the following:

• Walk with your family after work, using the time to catch up and spend quality time together.
• Walk with coworkers, instead of congregating in the break room.
• Walk any time someone gets on your nerves. It will help you rid your brain of those negative thoughts so that you can return to work focused.
• Walk every chance you get, even if that means parking in the space farthest from the grocery store, doing laps around your doctor's office as you wait for your appointment, or taking a quick stroll as dinner cooks in the oven.
• Walk with a friend instead of going out to eat or yakking on the phone.
• Schedule your powerwalks on your calendar.
• Think of walking as time to yourself away from life's other hassles.
• Get others involved. You'll be amazed at how far and how fast you can go when you have a juicy conversation to fuel the walk.
• Walk to a destination. Go on an "errand walk" where you hit the automated teller machine, pick up supplies from the hardware store, or return a borrowed book to a friend.
• Notice your surroundings. Try to recognize the birds you see and hear, or the trees and plants that you pass. If you're in a city, enjoy the window displays.
• Get a dog. Your dog just won't let you out of it.

ercise feel more taxing than it should. Your thighs might rub together and chafe; your joints may hurt under the weight of your body; you may simply have a tough time moving. Also, I hear from plenty of women and men who are too embarrassed to exercise at the gym in front of all of those hard bodies.

My 8 Minutes in the Morning powerwalking program addresses all of those concerns. After just 1 week of my 8 Minutes in the Morning program, many of these concerns will subside. Remember that my program not only helps you firm up from the outside but from the inside as well. That means you'll find confidence that you didn't know you had. And eventually, those fears of exercising in public will subside.

There are many reasons walking is extremely good for you. It will strengthen your heart and decrease your risk of various diseases, from heart disease to cancer to diabetes. Walking also helps when you're mad, sad, can't think straight, or when your mood is making you think about food.

The combination of getting your heart rate up and spending time outdoors melts stress away, making you more effective in everything you do. A 30-minute powerwalk leaves you relaxed and rejuvenated.

How many times have you decided not to do something or put your life on hold because you couldn't keep up or were too out of shape? Maybe your kids wanted to explore a nature trail or go to Disney World, and you weren't sure if you were up to it. Maybe a friend wanted to go on an all-day shopping spree at the mall, or your spouse suggested a romantic stroll on the boardwalk. My powerwalking plan will help you get in shape so that you will never have to use your body as an excuse again.

Studies show that most people who start powerwalking stick with it, compared to only half of those who try swimming, stair-stepping, or other forms of aerobic activity. That's probably because walking is one of the easiest activities to fit into a busy day (You can do it anywhere—even while waiting for your beeper to buzz you to your table at a packed restaurant.) Walking outside also gets you in touch with nature. The wind, fresh air, sunlight, natural colors, and animal life can all invigorate you.

If you're walking in the early morning or in the evening when it's dark, wear light-colored, reflective clothing to make yourself visible for oncoming cars. Carry a small flashlight in either hand. Attach cheap reflective tape to your clothes, or buy a reflective vest. And whenever you walk in the dark, try to do it with a companion. If the weather makes walking outdoors uncomfortable, or if safety is an issue, move indoors. Walk at a shopping mall or other large building. You can powerwalk through a grocery store, or even up and down hallways in a hotel. Investing in a treadmill for your home gym is a great way to make sure you can exercise every day, regardless.

What to Wear

The most important gear you need for walking is a sturdy pair of walking shoes. Those flimsy flats, loafers, or pumps that you wear to work simply aren't right for powerwalking. They'll slow you down, make you feel off-balance, and may make your legs ache. Even if you powerwalk in your work clothes, I suggest that you put on a pair of sneakers. You need good arch support and lots of cushioning. The more you weigh, the more support you'll need.

You can buy your sneakers at a department store or a sporting-goods store. They don't have to cost a lot of money, but they should fit well and feel good. It's best to try them on in the afternoon since your feet tend to swell during the day. Walk around the store and concentrate on how they feel. Does your heel slide up and down in the shoe? If so, you'll end up getting blisters. Do your toes feel pinched? Just imagine how they'll feel after 20 minutes of powerwalking.

Replace your shoes about every 6 months, or sooner. Pay attention to how your feet feel when you walk. As soon as they start to feel sore, replace your shoes. Also, your feet may shrink as you lose weight, which means that you'll need a new pair.

In addition to sneakers, you can buy an array of synthetic clothing that will wick moisture away from your body, keeping you dry and comfortable in both hot and cold weather. In the summer, light tops made of CoolMax and other synthetic materials keep you cool and dry and feel much lighter than cotton or any other natural fiber. In the winter, multiple layers of synthetic tights, long sleeve shirts, and jackets will block out the wind and keep you toasty without making you feel bulky.

How Far, How Fast?

When you first start walking, you might only be able to make it to the end of your driveway or to the end of your block. That's fine. You're out there and you're trying. And you just walked more than you walked yesterday. So give yourself a big pat on the back. After all, 1 minute or 5 minutes is better than no minutes at all.

For your first walk, go until you run out of breath or you start to tire. Build from there, increasing your time about 10 percent each week. Eventually, you want to be able to walk for 26 continuous minutes. (If you end up getting hooked and going much longer than 26 minutes, good for you! But I'm only asking you to do 26 minutes.) Three of those minutes should be a warmup and 3 of them a cooldown (see page 78). If you skip either of these, you risk injury. The warmup gets the fluid in your joints ready for the faster walking; the cooldown helps blood flow back to your heart instead of pooling in your legs, making you feel faint and weak.

Work on your distance first, then your intensity. You shouldn't pant and your legs shouldn't hurt. If you feel either, you're walking too fast or too far for your fitness level. Back off a little and then slowly add distance or intensity. If you rate your effort on a scale from 1 to 10, it should fall somewhere between 6 and 8. That's your fat-burning zone. You'll feel better in that zone as well as reap the most benefits from the exercise.

How to Walk Well

Powerwalking with proper posture will save your knees, especially if you still have a lot of weight to lose. Walking with good form will also increase the number of calories you burn and make your walk more enjoyable. You want walking to be a *total-body experience*, not just something that involves your legs, so make an effort to use your upper body, which will increase your caloric burn.

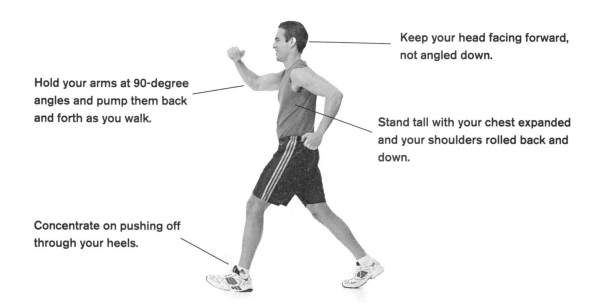

Hold your arms at 90-degree angles and pump them back and forth as you walk.

Keep your head facing forward, not angled down.

Stand tall with your chest expanded and your shoulders rolled back and down.

Concentrate on pushing off through your heels.

After-Walk Stretches

I recommend that you do the following stretches. It's always best to stretch after your walk, when the muscles are already warm.

Calf Stretch: Stand 2 to 3 feet away from a wall. Place your palms on the wall with your left foot in front of the other, about 2 feet apart. Lean into the wall with your left leg bent and your right leg straight. Feel the stretch in your calf. Hold for 20 seconds and then switch legs.

Deep Calf Stretch: Stand 2 to 3 feet away from a wall. Place your palms on the wall with your left foot in front of the other, about 2 feet apart. Lean into the wall with your left leg bent and your left leg straight, then bend your right leg so that the stretch moves to a different area on your calf. Hold for 20 seconds and then switch legs.

Hamstring Stretch: Lie on your back on a mat with your legs bent. Bring your left leg up and thread a towel around your thigh. Hold your thigh at about a 90-degree angle (if you can). Straighten your leg as much as possible. Hold for 20 seconds and then switch legs.

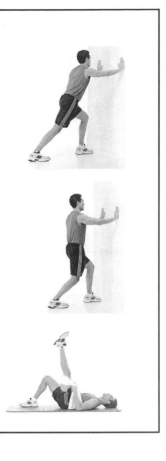

Treadmill Recommendations

Many of you have emailed me and asked what home treadmill I personally recommend for powerwalking. Well, www.stairmaster.com showcases my favorite treadmill the Club Track 612 Plus. You can adapt all your powerwalking to this excellent deluxe system with great comfort and safety. If you have a tighter budget, then visit www.nautilus.com and check out the new Nautilus NTR line. Regardless, you will love both of these great treadmills.

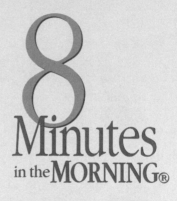

PART FOUR

Resources

The Easy Way
to Eat Fat to Get Fit

The following pages will be invaluable to you as you begin and maintain the 8 Minutes in the Morning way of life. Use these pages for quick reference and to guide your daily food choices. Everything's here:

- A comprehensive Food List, including the number of boxes each item equals
- Exciting and simple-to-make recipes to help you get those veggies into your meals effortlessly
- The very important Quick Start menu plan, which makes your first week of eating healthier a "no-brainer"
- The Eating Cards, your insurance policy for eating right every day

There are two blank Eating Cards on page 234 for you to copy, cut out, staple together, and carry with you. Make four copies to get enough cards for a week, plus one extra. Give the extra to a friend and introduce her to a new 8 Minutes in the Morning life, too!

Food List

H ere is everything you need to know about the foods you can eat and the proper serving sizes. This is what each box on your Eating Card equals. These (approximate) caloric values have been developed by the American Dietetic Association.

Fat = 45 calories

Protein = 75 calories

Complex Carbohydrate = 80 calories

Dairy = 90 calories

Vegetables = 25 calories

Fruit = 60 calories

Treats and Cravings = 30 calories

Fat Unless otherwise specified, cross off 1 Fat box on your Eating Card for each specified amount.

Preferred Fats

Almond butter (1 tablespoon)—
 PLUS 1 Protein box

Almonds, raw (6)

Avocado (⅛ medium)

Cashews (6)

Flax oil (1 teaspoon or 4 capsules)

Oil-based salad dressing
 (1 tablespoon)

Olive oil (1 teaspoon)

Olives (10 small or 5 large)

Peanut butter (2 teaspoons)
 —PLUS 1 Protein box

Peanuts (10)

Pecans (4 halves)

Pumpkin seeds (1 tablespoon)

Sesame seeds (1 tablespoon)

Soy mayonnaise (1 tablespoon)

Sunflower seeds (1 tablespoon)

Tahini paste (2 teaspoons)

Fats to Minimize

Butter, reduced-calorie
 (1 tablespoon)

Butter, stick (1 teaspoon)

Butter, whipped (2 teaspoons)

Coconut (2 tablespoons)

Corn oil (1 teaspoon)

Cream cheese (1 tablespoon)

Cream cheese, reduced-calorie
 (2 tablespoons)

Half-and-half (2 tablespoons)

Lard (1 teaspoon)

Mayonnaise (1 teaspoon)

Mayonnaise, reduced-calorie (1 tablespoon)

Shortening (1 teaspoon)

Sour cream (2 tablespoons)

Sour cream, reduced-calorie (3 tablespoons)

Protein

Unless otherwise specified, check off 1 Protein box on your Eating Card for each specified amount. Higher-fat selections will require you to check off 1 or 2 Fat boxes in addition to the Protein box. Meat protein sources are based on cooked portions; raw meat will shrink when cooking. A 4-ounce raw chicken breast will shrink to 3 ounces when cooked.

Preferred Proteins

•Beans

Black, cooked (½ cup)
Chickpeas, cooked (½ cup)
Hummus (¼ cup)—PLUS 1 Fat box
Kidney, cooked (½ cup)
Lentil, cooked (½ cup)
Lima, cooked (½ cup)
Pinto, cooked (½ cup)
Refried, fat-added (⅓ cup)—PLUS 1 Fat box
Refried, fat-free (⅓ cup)
Split peas, cooked (½ cup)
White, cooked (½ cup)

•Eggs

Egg, whole (1)
Egg substitute (¼ cup)
Egg whites (3)

•Poultry

Chicken or turkey, white meat without skin
 (1 ounce)
Chicken or turkey, dark meat with skin
 (1 ounce)—PLUS 1 Fat box

•Seafood

Fish, canned

Salmon, packed in water (¼ cup)
Sardines, packed in water (2 medium)

White tuna, packed
 in water (¼ cup)

Fish, fresh or frozen

Flounder (1 ounce)
Fried fish (1 ounce)—PLUS 1 Fat box
Mahi mahi (1 ounce)
Salmon (1 ounce)
Sea bass (1 ounce)
Sole (1 ounce)
Swordfish (1 ounce)
Tuna (1 ounce)

Shellfish

Clams (2 ounces)
Crab (2 ounces)
Crawfish (2 ounces)
Lobster (2 ounces)
Oysters (6 medium)
Scallops (2 ounces)
Shrimp (2 ounces)

•Soy Products

Soybeans, cooked (½ cup)
Soy burger (½ burger)
Soy cheese (1 ounce)
Soy hot dog (1)
Soy milk, fortified, 1% or fat-free (8 ounces)
Texturized soy protein (1 teaspoon or 1 ounce)
Tofu (½ cup)

Proteins to Minimize

•Red Meats

Bacon (1 slice)—PLUS 1 Fat box

Goat (1 ounce)

Ham, smoked or fresh (1 ounce)

Hot dog, beef, pork, or both (1)—PLUS 2 Fat boxes

Lamb shank or shoulder (1 ounce)

London broil (1 ounce)

Round steak (1 ounce)

Sirloin steak (1 ounce)

Skirt steak (1 ounce)

Tenderloin (1 ounce)

Veal chop or roast (1 ounce)

Complex Carbohydrates
Unless otherwise specified, check off 1 Complex Carbohydrate box on your Eating Card for each specified amount. Higher-fat selections will require you to check off 1 or 2 Fat boxes in addition to the Complex Carbohydrate box. If you can't find a particular complex carbohydrate listed, check off one box for every ½-cup serving of cereal, grain, pasta, or starchy vegetable. Remember that whole grain products are ideal, but if you eat out or are traveling and whole grain products are not available, non–whole grain versions are acceptable in moderation.

Preferred Carbohydrates

•Whole Grain Breads

Bagel (½ of a 2-ounce bagel)

Bread (1 ounce or 1 slice)

English muffin (½)

Hamburger roll (½)

Nan (bread from India) (¼ of 8" x 2" loaf)

Pita, 6-inch (½)

Roll, dinner (1 small)

Tortilla, corn, 6-inch (1)

Tortilla, flour, 7-inch (1)

Waffle, fat-free (1)

•Whole Grain Cereals and Grains

Barley, cooked (½ cup)

Basmati rice, cooked (⅓ cup)

Brown rice, cooked (⅓ cup)

Buckwheat (Kasha), cooked (½ cup)

Bulgur, cooked (½ cup)

Cereal, cold, sweetened (½ cup)

Cereal, cold, unsweetened (¾ cup)

Cereal, hot (½ cup)

Couscous, cooked (½ cup)

Granola, low-fat (½ cup)

Hominy grits, cooked (½ cup)

Jasmine rice, cooked (⅓ cup)

Wheat germ (3 tablespoons)

Wild rice, cooked (⅓ cup)

•Whole Grain Flour

Cornstarch (2 tablespoons)

Matzo meal (⅓ cup)

Whole wheat flour, all-purpose (2½ tablespoons)

•Whole Grain Pasta

Spelt and millet, cooked spaghetti noodles (½ cup)

Whole grain, cooked spaghetti noodles (½ cup)
Whole wheat, cooked spaghetti noodles (½ cup)

Carbohydrates to Minimize

•Starchy Vegetables

Corn (½ cup)
Corn on the cob (6-inch ear)
French fries (10)—PLUS 1 Fat box
Green peas (½ cup)
Potato, baked (1 small)
Potato, instant (⅓ cup)

Potato, mashed (½ cup)
Pumpkin (½ cup)
Sweet potato (⅓ cup)
Winter squash, acorn or butternut (¾ cup)
Yucca root (cassava), boiled (½ cup)

•Crackers

Matzo (¾ ounce)
Melba toast (4 slices)
Oyster crackers (24)
Saltine crackers (6)
Whole wheat crackers (2–5)

Dairy
Each serving from dairy contains 90 calories. For portions of cheese that have 56 to 80 calories per ounce, check off 1 Dairy and 1 Fat box per ounce unless otherwise specified. For cheese portions that are whole-milk varieties (more than 80 calories per ounce), check off 1 Dairy and 2 Fat boxes unless otherwise specified.

Cheese (55 calories or less per ounce)

American (1 ounce)
Cheddar (1 ounce)
Cottage, low-fat or fat-free (¼ cup)
Feta (1 ounce)
Monterey Jack (1 ounce)
Muenster (1 ounce)
Parmesan, grated (1 tablespoon)
Provolone (1 ounce)
Ricotta, low-fat or fat-free (¼ cup)
Soy, all varieties (1 ounce)
Swiss (1 ounce)

Milk Products

Lactose-free milk, low-fat or fat-free (8 ounces)
Milk, 1% or fat-free (8 ounces)
Milk, whole (8 ounces)—PLUS 2 Fat boxes
Nonfat dry milk (⅓ cup)
Soy milk, fortified, 1% or fat-free (8 ounces)
Yogurt, frozen, low-fat or nonfat (½ cup)
Yogurt, low-fat or nonfat, flavored (8 ounces)—
   PLUS 1 Fruit box and 2 Treats and Cravings
   boxes
Yogurt, low-fat or nonfat, plain (8 ounces)
Yogurt, whole milk, plain (8 ounces)—PLUS
   check off 2 Fat boxes

Vegetables

Vegetables There are two kinds of vegetables in this section: limited ones, which are higher in calories, and unlimited ones. You may have as many of the unlimited vegetables as you wish. You don't have to cross off any Veggie boxes on your Eating Card for the unlimited ones. Vegetables that are high in starch do not appear on this list; they are on the Complex Carbohydrates list.

For each specified "Limited Vegetable" amount, check off 1 Veggie box on your Eating Card. All servings are 1 cup raw or ½ cup cooked, unless otherwise specified.

Limited Vegetables

Artichoke, (½ medium)
Asparagus
Beet greens
Beets
Bell peppers
Broccoli
Brussels sprouts
Carrots
Cauliflower
Chayote (squash)
Collard greens
Eggplant
Green beans
Kale
Leeks
Mung bean sprouts
Onions
Parsnips
Pea pods
Pickles (1½ large)
Rutabaga
Sauerkraut
Seaweed, raw
Snow peas

String beans
Tomatillo, raw (1 medium)
Tomato (1 medium)
Tomato paste (3 tablespoons)
Tomato puree (½ cup)
Tomato sauce (½ cup)
Tomatoes, canned (½ cup)
Turnips
Vegetable soup, fat-free, low-sodium (½ cup)

Unlimited Vegetables

Alfalfa sprouts
Cabbage
Celery
Cucumber
Garlic
Green onions
Jalapeño and other hot peppers
Lettuce, all types
Mushrooms
Radishes
Spinach
Watercress
Zucchini

Fruits
Unless otherwise specified, check off 1 Fruit box on your Eating Card for each specified amount. If you can't find a particular fruit listed, check off 1 box for every small to medium fresh fruit, ½ cup canned fruit, or ¼ cup dried fruit.

Limited Fruit

Apple, green or red (1 medium)
Apple juice (½ cup)
Applesauce, unsweetened (½ cup)
Apricots (4)
Banana (½ medium)
Blackberries (¾ cup)
Blueberries (¾ cup)
Cantaloupe (⅓ melon or 1 cup cubed)
Cherries (12 large)
Cranberry juice (½ cup)
Fruit cocktail (½ cup)
Grapefruit (½)
Grapefruit juice (½ cup)
Grapes, green or red (12)
Honeydew (⅓ melon or 1 cup cubed)
Kiwifruit (1 large)
Orange (1 medium)
Orange juice (½ cup)
Peach (1 medium)
Pear, green (1 small)
Pineapple, canned, packed in juice (⅓ cup)
Plums (2 medium)
Prunes (2)
Raisins (2 tablespoons)
Raspberries (1 cup)
Strawberries (1 cup)
Watermelon (1 cup cubed)

Unlimited Fruit

Lemons
Limes

Treats and Cravings
Check off 1 Treats and Cravings box on your Eating Card for each specified amount.

Angel food cake, unfrosted (1/12 of cake)
Animal crackers (8)
Brownie (2" square)—PLUS 1 Fat box
Cake with frosting (1" square)—PLUS 1 Fat box
Chicken rice soup, prepared with water (½ cup)
Chocolate candies (6 pieces or 1 ounce)—PLUS 1
  Treats and Cravings box and 2 Fat boxes
Cocoa powder (1 tablespoon)
Cookie with cream filling (2 small)—PLUS 1 Fat box
Cranberry sauce (¼ cup)
Cupcake with frosting (1)—PLUS 1 Fat box
Doughnut (½)—PLUS 1 Fat box
Fat-free cookies (2 small)
Fat-free potato chips (15 to 20)
Fat-free tortilla chips (15 to 20)
Fortune cookie (1)
Fruit juice frozen bar (1 bar)
Gelatin (½ cup)

Gingersnaps (3)
Graham cracker (2½" square)
Granola bar (1)—PLUS 1 Fat box
Gumdrops (8 small)
Hard candy (1)
Ice cream (½ cup)—PLUS 2 Fat boxes
Ice cream, light (½ cup)—PLUS 1 Fat box
Jelly beans (7)
Licorice twist (1)
Marshmallow (1 large)
Milk chocolate bar (1.6 ounce)—PLUS 1 Complex
  Carbohydrate box and 3 Fat boxes
Oatmeal cookie (1 medium)—PLUS 1 Complex Car-
  bohydrate box and 1 Fat box

Pancake syrup, low-calorie (1 tablespoon)
Popcorn, nonfat (1 cup)
Potato chips, fat-free (6) with salsa (½ tablespoon)
Pretzels, unsalted (10 small sticks)
Rice cakes, mini (2)
Saltine crackers, unsalted (6)
Sorbet (¼ cup)
Table sugar (1 teaspoon)—PLUS 1 Complex Carbohy-
  drate box
Tortilla chips (6 to 12)—PLUS 2 Fat boxes
Tea, herbal, with 1 teaspoon honey (1 cup)
Vanilla wafers (5)—PLUS 1 Fat box
Whipped topping, nondairy, fat-free (3 tablespoons)

Alcohol Check off 2 Fat boxes for each of the specified amounts.

Beer (12 ounces)—PLUS 1 Complex
  Carbohydrate box
Beer, light (12 ounces)

Liquor (1½ ounces)
Wine (5 ounces)

Fast Foods Busy, on-the-go lifestyles often means resorting to quick meals, whether it's a frozen dinner or something from a fast-food burger place. I recommend that you make your own meals, but here's a sampling of what to check off on your Eating Cards for various meal combinations when you're short on time.

Burritos with chicken (2): 2 Fat boxes; 2 Protein boxes; 4 Complex Carbohydrate boxes
Chicken nuggets (6): 1 Fat box; 2 Protein boxes; 1 Complex Carbohydrate box
Fish sandwich with tartar sauce (1): 3 Fat boxes; 1 Protein box; 3 Complex Carbohydrate boxes
French fries (20 to 25): 2 Fat boxes; 2 Complex Carbohydrate boxes
Fried chicken breast and wing (1 each): 2 Fat boxes; 4 Protein boxes; 1 Complex Carbohydrate box
Hamburger, regular (1): 2 Fat boxes; 2 Protein boxes; 2 Complex Carbohydrate boxes

Hot dog with bun (1): 1 Fat box; 1 Protein box; 1 Complex Carbohydrate box

Pizza, thin crust with cheese (3 small slices): 1 Fat box; 2 Protein boxes; 2 Complex Carbohydrate boxes

Pizza with meat topping (3 small slices): 2 Fat boxes; 2 Protein boxes; 2 Complex Carbohydrate boxes

Salisbury steak with gravy frozen dinner (11 ounces): 2 Fat boxes; 2 Protein boxes; 2 Complex Carbohydrate boxes

Submarine sandwich (6 inch): 1 Fat box; 2 Protein boxes; 3 Complex Carbohydrate boxes; 1 Veggie box

Taco, hard shell (6 ounces): 2 Fat boxes; 2 Protein boxes; 2 Complex Carbohydrate boxes

Taco, soft shell (3 ounces): 1 Fat box; 1 Protein box; 1 Complex Carbohydrate box

Turkey with gravy, mashed potatoes, and dressing frozen dinner (11 ounces): 2 Fat boxes; 2 Protein boxes; 2 Complex Carbohydrate boxes

For an extended food list, visit www.JorgeCruise.com/foodlist.

Bonus Items Don't check off any boxes.

Carbonated or sparkling water (add lime or lemon for great taste!)

Club soda

Condiments—Mustard, ketchup, barbecue sauce, steak sauce, fat-free salad dressing (3 tablespoons per day)

Diet soda with aspartame and saccharin (2 per day)

Green or herbal tea or decaffeinated coffee (2 per day)

Nonstick cooking spray

Salsas—Tabasco sauce, hot-pepper sauce, pico de gallo, picante sauce

Stevia (a natural sweetener available at all health food stores)

A Week of Eating Fat to Get Fit

The following menu contains exactly the number of calories and the breakdown of foods that you should eat during your *first week* of your 8 Minutes in the Morning program. I strongly urge you use this "quick-start" menu as a guide for week 1. For weeks 2, 3, 4, and beyond, you will need to eat the appropriate number of calories on the Eating Card System (see page 70). You can move some food portions to other meals if you like; the only hard rule is that you can't move your fat. You must have fat with each main meal. You can also repeat or "mix and match" the breakfasts, lunches, or dinners as desired.

Day 1

Breakfast: 3 scrambled egg whites, 1 slice toast with 1 teaspoon flax or olive oil, 1 cup soy milk, ½ grapefruit, 1 cup green tea or decaffeinated coffee (1 Protein, 1 Complex Carb, 1 Fat, 1 Dairy, 1 Fruit)

Lunch: 1 soy hot dog on a bun with mustard and/or ketchup, ½ cup corn, large mixed-greens salad with 1 teaspoon flax oil, ½ cup frozen low-fat yogurt, 1 licorice twist (1 Protein, 2 Complex Carbohydrates, 2 Veggies, 1 Fat, 1 Dairy, 1 Treat/Craving)

Dinner: ½ BLT sandwich with avocado (1 slice bread with 1 ounce turkey bacon, iceberg lettuce, tomato, and ⅛ avocado), 1 cup tomato soup, 1 diet soda (1 Complex Carb, 1 Protein, 2 Veggies, 1 Fat)

Snack: 1 cup air-popped popcorn (1 Treat/Craving)

Day 2

Breakfast: ¼ cup whole grain cereal with 1 cup soy milk, 1 hard-boiled egg, 1 teaspoon flax oil, 1 small banana or ½ medium banana, 1 cup green tea or decaffeinated coffee (1 Complex Carb, 1 Dairy, 1 Protein, 1 Fat, 1 Fruit)

Lunch: 1 cup lentil soup with 1 teaspoon flax oil added, medium whole grain roll, large plate of steamed vegetables, ½ cup frozen low-fat yogurt, 1 fortune cookie, 1 glass club soda (1 Protein, 1 Fat, 1 Complex Carb, 2 Veggies, 1 Dairy, 1 Treat/Craving)

Dinner: Tuna pasta salad (¼ cup white tuna (water-packed) mixed with 1 tablespoon reduced-calorie mayonnaise, 2 tablespoons chopped onion and pickle, and ½ cup cooked penne pasta over lettuce), 1 small (6-inch) corn-on-the-cob, large plate of steamed vegetables, 1 sparkling water with lemon (1 Protein, 1 Fat, 2 Complex Carbs, 2 Veggies)

Snack: 8 animal crackers (1 Treat/Craving)

Day 3

Breakfast: ½ toasted English muffin with 1 teaspoon flax oil, 3-egg-white omelet with vegetables, 1 glass soy milk, 1 apple, 1 cup green tea or decaffeinated coffee (1 Complex Carb, 1 Fat, 1 Protein, 1 Veggie, 1 Dairy, 1 Fruit)

Lunch: ½ turkey sandwich (1 slice bread with 1 ounce white-meat turkey, lettuce, tomato, and mustard), 1 cup vegetable soup with 1 teaspoon flax oil added, ½ cup frozen low-fat yogurt, 1 diet soda (1 Complex Carb, 1 Protein, 2 Veggies, 1 Fat, 1 Dairy)

Dinner: Lettuce wrap (1 ounce white-meat chicken, ½ cup brown rice, and salsa wrapped in a large iceberg lettuce leaf), large mixed-greens salad with 1 teaspoon of flax oil, 4 whole wheat crackers, 1 large marshmallow, 1 glass sparkling water with lemon (1 Protein, 2 Complex Carbs, 1 Veggie, 1 Fat, 1 Treat/Craving)

Snack: 2 fat-free cookies (1 Treat/Craving)

Day 4

Breakfast: ½ cup low-fat granola mixed with ½ cup yogurt and ¾ cup fresh fruit salad, 3 egg whites scrambled with 1 teaspoon flax oil, 1 cup green tea or decaffeinated coffee (1 Complex Carb, 1 Dairy, 1 Fruit, 1 Protein, 1 Fat)

Lunch: Chicken baked potato (1 small baked potato topped with 1 ounce cubed sautéed chicken breast, 1 ounce cheese, and salsa), large plate of steamed vegetables with 1 teaspoon flax oil, ½ cup gelatin, 1 glass club soda (1 Complex Carb, 1 Protein, 1 Dairy, 2 Veggies, 1 Fat, 1 Treat/Craving)

Dinner: Pasta with meat sauce (½ cup cooked pasta with 1 ounce cooked ground turkey breast, tomato sauce, and garlic), large mixed-greens salad with 1 teaspoon flax oil, 1 dinner roll, 1 diet soda (2 Complex Carbs, 1 Protein, 2 Veggies, 1 Fat)

Snack: 1 cup air-popped popcorn (1 Treat/Craving)

Day 5

Breakfast: ½ cup oatmeal with 1 cup soy milk and 1 teaspoon flax oil, 1 hard-boiled egg, ½ small bagel, 1 cup green tea or decaffeinated coffee (2 Complex Carbs, 1 Dairy, 1 Fat, 1 Protein)

Lunch: 1 cup chili with 1 teaspoon flax oil added, 1 whole grain tortilla, large plate of steamed vegetables, ½ cup low-fat frozen yogurt, 1 licorice twist, 1 glass sparkling water with lemon (1 Protein, 1 Fat, 1 Complex Carb, 2 Veggies, 1 Dairy, 1 Treat/Craving)

Dinner: Fajitas (1 ounce cooked chicken breast or beef, ¼ cup onions, and peppers sautéed with Pam or water, then wrapped in a tortilla with tomato, lettuce, and 2 tablespoons guacamole), ½ cup fruit salad, 1 diet soda (1 Protein, 2 Veggies, 1 Complex Carb, 1 Fat, 1 Fruit)

Snack: Graham crackers (2½"-square) (1 Treat/Craving)

Day 6

Breakfast: 1 slice toast with 2 teaspoons peanut or almond butter, 1 ounce cooked ham, ½ cup plain low-fat yogurt mixed with ½ cup strawberries, 1 cup green tea or de-caffeinated coffee (1 Complex Carb, 1 Fat, 1 Protein, 1 Dairy, 1 Fruit)

Lunch: Tuna pita (¼ cup white tuna (water-packed) mixed with 1 tablespoon low-calorie mayonnaise spooned into ½ pita with lettuce and tomato), 1 cup vegetable soup, ½ cup frozen low-fat yogurt, 2 tablespoons raisins, 1 diet soda (1 Protein, 1 Fat, 1 Complex Carb, 2 Veggies, 1 Dairy, 1 Treat/Craving)

Dinner: 1 ounce grilled salmon with grilled onions and garlic, ½ cup rice, large green salad with 1 tablespoon oil-based dressing, 8 small gumdrops, 1 glass club soda (1 Protein, 1 Complex Carb, 2 Veggies, 1 Fat, 1 Treat/Craving)

Snack: ½ small bagel (1 Complex Carb)

Day 7

Breakfast: Breakfast burrito (1 small whole wheat tortilla filled with 3 scrambled egg whites, 1 ounce cheese, 1 teaspoon flax oil, and salsa), 1 apple, 1 cup green tea or decaffeinated coffee (1 Complex Carb, 1 Protein, 1 Dairy, 1 Fat, 1 Fruit)

Lunch: Turkey melt (1 slice whole wheat toast topped with 1 ounce white-meat turkey and 1 slice soy or regular cheese then broiled for 2 minutes), large mixed-greens salad with 1 teaspoon flax oil, 1 licorice twist, 1 diet soda (1 Complex Carb, 1 Protein, 1 Dairy, 1 Veggie, 1 Fat, 1 Treat/Craving)

Dinner: Chinese stir-fry (1 ounce chicken breast or beef, 2 cups vegetables stir-fried with water, pepper, and low-sodium soy sauce over ½ cup brown rice), large mixed-greens salad with 1 teaspoon flax oil, 1 dinner roll, 1 glass sparkling water with lemon (1 Protein, 3 Veggies, 2 Complex Carbs, 1 Fat)

Snack: 1 cup air-popped popcorn (1 Treat/Craving)

Jorge's Recipes

H ere are some great healthy recipes, most chock-full of veggies, to help keep you going strong in weeks 2, 3, 4, and beyond of the Eat Fat to Get Fit program.

Chinese Veggie Stir-Fry
(1 Protein box, 2 Veggie boxes)

½ cup low-sodium soy sauce
½ cup water
½ cup cubed tofu (optional)
½ cup chopped white onion
4 cloves garlic, minced
½ cup broccoli florets

1 tablespoon minced fresh ginger
½ cup sliced carrot
½ cup sliced mushroom
½ cup snow pea pods
½ cup diced celery
¼ cup sliced water chestnuts

In a wok or large skillet, heat the soy sauce and water over high heat. Add the tofu (if using), onion, and garlic. Sauté for 2 minutes. Add the broccoli, ginger, and carrots. Sauté for 4 minutes. Add the mushrooms, pea pods, celery, and water chestnuts. Continue to stir-fry until the vegetables are al dente. You may add more water or soy sauce, if desired. *Makes 6 servings*

Asian Broccoli and Cauliflower Salad
(1 Veggie box, 1½ Fat boxes)

3 cups broccoli florets
3 cups cauliflower florets
1 tablespoon olive oil
2 tablespoons sesame oil

4 tablespoons low-sodium soy sauce
¾ cup chopped scallions
4 cloves garlic, minced

In a large saucepan, blanch the broccoli and cauliflower in 2 quarts of boiling water for 3 minutes. Drain in a colander and rinse with cold water. Combine the olive oil, sesame oil, soy sauce, scallions, and garlic in a medium bowl. Mix in the broccoli and cauliflower. Chill before serving. *Makes 6 servings*

Cucumber-Tomato Salad
(1 Veggie box)

4 plum tomatoes, chopped
3 cucumbers, peeled, seeded, and chopped

1 tablespoon olive oil
Salt and pepper, to taste

In a medium bowl, mix the tomatoes, cucumbers, and oil. Season with the salt and pepper. Chill before serving. *Makes 6 servings*

Grilled Chicken Salad
(2 Protein boxes, 3 Veggie boxes, 1 Fat box)

2 ounces grilled chicken breast
2 cups lettuce
½ cup diced tomato

½ cup shredded carrot
1 tablespoon dressing

In a large bowl, toss together the chicken, lettuce, tomato, and carrot. Add the dressing and mix well. *Makes 1 serving*

Pasta with Veggies
(2 Complex Carbohydrate boxes, 2 Veggie boxes, 1 Fat box)

1 tablespoon olive oil
½ cup chopped tomato
½ cup sliced zucchini
½ cup sliced mushroom

½ cup chopped basil
2 cloves garlic, minced
Freshly ground black pepper, to taste
1 cup cooked whole grain pasta

Heat the oil in a large skillet. Sauté the tomato, zucchini, mushroom, basil, and garlic over medium-high heat until tender. Season with the pepper. Serve the pasta topped with the vegetables. *Makes 1 serving*

Egg-White Scramble
(1 Protein box, 1 Veggie box)

¼ cup chopped tomato
¼ cup chopped onion
¼ cup chopped mushroom

¼ cup chopped zucchini
3 egg whites
¼ cup salsa

Coat a medium skillet with cooking spray. Scramble the tomato, onion, mushroom, and zucchini into the egg whites. Top with the salsa. *Makes 1 serving*

Three-Bean Salad
(1 Protein box, 2 Veggie boxes, 1 Fat box)

¼ cup cooked chickpeas
¼ cup cooked kidney beans
½ cup steamed green beans
¼ cup chopped red onion

1 teaspoon olive oil
1 tomato, diced
1 teaspoon balsamic vinegar
1 cup chopped lettuce

In a medium bowl, toss the chickpeas, kidney beans, and green beans with the onion, oil, tomato, and vinegar. Serve over the lettuce. *Makes 1 serving*

Variation: Use canned mixed beans.

Roasted Chicken
(2 Protein boxes)

2 ounces skinless, boneless chicken breast

1 tablespoon chopped fresh sage
1 tablespoon chopped fresh rosemary

Preheat the oven to 350°F. Coat the chicken with cooking spray. Sprinkle evenly with the sage and rosemary. Roast for 45 minutes or until a thermometer inserted in the thickest portion registers 160°F and the juices run clear. *Makes 1 serving*

Burrito

(1 Complex Carbohydrate box, 2 Protein boxes, 1 Veggie box)

½ cup fat-free refried beans
½ cup chopped lettuce
1 ounce shredded soy cheese

1 whole wheat tortilla (7-inch)
½ cup salsa

Wrap the refried beans, lettuce, and cheese in the tortilla. Place the tortilla in a small cast-iron skillet and heat over medium heat until both sides are slightly brown. Remove and top with the salsa. *Makes 1 serving*

Pita Pizza

(2 Complex Carbohydrate boxes, 1 Protein box, 1 Veggie box, 1 Fat box)

1 teaspoon olive oil
½ cup chopped steamed broccoli
½ cup chopped tomato
¼ cup diced fresh basil

1 teaspoon minced garlic
1 whole wheat pita
1 ounce shredded mozzarella soy cheese

Preheat the broiler. Heat the oil in a medium skillet. Sauté the broccoli, tomato, basil, and garlic over medium-high heat. Spoon the mixture onto the pita and sprinkle with the cheese. Broil for 1 to 2 minutes, or until the cheese melts. *Makes 1 serving*

Tuna Melt

(1 Complex Carbohydrate box, 2 Protein boxes, 1 Fat box)

¼ cup water-packed white tuna
1 tablespoon chopped red onion
1 tablespoon chopped pickle
1 tablespoon reduced-calorie or soy mayonnaise

1 slice whole wheat bread
1 ounce Cheddar soy cheese

Preheat the broiler. Mix the tuna with the onion, pickle, and mayonnaise. Spoon the mixture onto the bread and top with the cheese. Broil for 1 to 2 minutes, or until the cheese melts. *Makes 1 serving*

Hot Veggie Pita Sandwich

(2 Complex Carbohydrate boxes, 1 Protein box, 3 Veggie boxes)

- 3 cups chopped vegetables
- ¼ cup chopped onion
- 1 teaspoon minced garlic
- 1 whole wheat pita
- 1 ounce shredded soy cheese

Coat a large skillet with cooking spray. Sauté the vegetables, onion, and garlic over medium-high heat. Slice the pita in half and stuff each half with the mixture. Add the cheese. *Makes 1 serving*

Salmon Salad

(1 Protein box, 2 Veggie boxes, 1 Fat box)

- 2 ounces grilled or canned salmon
- ¼ cup chopped red onion
- ¼ cup chopped tomato
- ¼ cup shredded carrot
- ¼ cup sliced mushroom
- 1 cup chopped lettuce
- 1 tablespoon reduced-calorie dressing

In a medium bowl, toss the salmon, onion, tomato, carrot, and mushroom with the lettuce. Add the dressing and mix well. *Makes 1 serving*

Chicken Fajitas

(2 Complex Carbohydrate boxes, 1 Protein box, 1½ Veggie boxes)

- 2 ounces sliced chicken breast
- ½ cup sliced onion
- ½ cup sliced red bell pepper
- ½ cup sliced green bell pepper
- Freshly ground black pepper, to taste
- 2 whole wheat or corn tortillas (7-inch)

Coat a medium skillet with cooking spray. Sauté the chicken, onion, and red and green bell peppers over medium-high heat. Season with the black pepper. Spoon the mixture into the tortillas and roll up to enclose the filling. *Makes 2 servings*

The Eat Fat to Get Fit Eating Card System

Eating the best kinds of food in the right amounts is key to being successful in your weight-loss journey. I have created Eating Cards to take all the guesswork out of it for you.

First, draw a thick rule over the dotted line next to your calorie selection (see page 70). In the sample card, the line is to the right of the quick start. The boxes to the left are the servings of each food you can enjoy each day. Mark off the boxes corresponding to the type and amount of food you eat. Here, the person has eaten the recommended breakfast and lunch from the Quick Start menu (on page 219) plus 5 glasses of water. The unchecked boxes show what she can eat for dinner and any snacks. When all the boxes are checked off, you are done eating for the rest of the day.

I've included two master Eating Cards on page 234. Photocopy them and keep them with you all the time. It's easier to mark them as the day goes on, so you don't forget. Just cut the cards on the dotted lines, stack them, and staple them in the upper left-hand corner to make a little booklet. You can put the booklet into an old checkbook cover to protect it and make it very convenient to use!

Your Eating Card System

Draw a thick line over the dotted line to the right of your calorie selection. Everything to the left is your daily food intake.

Date: _____

	Quick Start (Week 1) ◄	1,200 ◄	1,400 ◄	1,600 ◄	1,800 ◄	2,000 ◄
Fats	☒ ☒ ☐	☐		☐	☐ ☐	☐
Proteins	☒ ☒ ☐	☐	☐	☐		☐
Complex Carbs	☒ ☒ ☒ ☐		☐	☐	☐	☐
Dairy	☒ ☒					
Veggies	☒ ☒ ☐ ☐	☐	☐			
Fruits	☒					
Treats/Cravings	☒ ☐				☐	
Water	☒ ☒ ☒ ☒ ☒ ☐ ☐ ☐	www.jorgecruise.com				

Instructions for blank Eating Cards: Make four copies for each week. Cut on the dotted lines, then stack and staple in the upper left-hand corner. Keep them with you at all times.

Your Eating Card System

Draw a thick line over the dotted line to the right of your calorie selection. Everything to the left is your daily food intake.

Date: _____

	Quick Start (Week 1)	1,200	1,400	1,600	1,800	2,000
Fats	☐ ☐ ☐	☐		☐	☐ ☐	☐
Proteins	☐ ☐ ☐	☐	☐	☐		☐
Complex Carbs	☐ ☐ ☐ ☐		☐	☐	☐	☐
Dairy	☐ ☐					
Veggies	☐ ☐ ☐ ☐	☐	☐			
Fruits	☐					
Treats/Cravings	☐ ☐				☐	
Water	☐ ☐ ☐ ☐ ☐ ☐ ☐ ☐	www.jorgecruise.com				

Draw a thick line over the dotted line to the right of your calorie selection. Everything to the left is your daily food intake.

Date: _____

	Quick Start (Week 1)	1,200	1,400	1,600	1,800	2,000
Fats	☐ ☐ ☐	☐		☐	☐ ☐	☐
Proteins	☐ ☐ ☐	☐	☐	☐		☐
Complex Carbs	☐ ☐ ☐ ☐		☐	☐	☐	☐
Dairy	☐ ☐					
Veggies	☐ ☐ ☐ ☐	☐	☐			
Fruits	☐					
Treats/Cravings	☐ ☐				☐	
Water	☐ ☐ ☐ ☐ ☐ ☐ ☐ ☐	www.jorgecruise.com				

ALL NEW!

The Cruise Control™ Secret

Jorge Cruise's Secret to Eliminating Emotional Eating

A re you ready to take your 8 Minutes in the Morning weight loss plan up a notch? Are you ready to discover how to make your weight loss happen even faster and easier?

In the next few pages you will learn my all-new secret for eliminating the number one roadblock to your long-term weight loss success: *emotional eating*. What exactly is emotional eating? It's the trigger that causes you to eat when you are not hungry. It's the catalyst that induces you to eat for reasons other than to provide your body with energy or with the necessary nutrients to build new tissues. Instead, emotional eating encourages you to use food to improve your mood. If, when you feel sad, depressed, stressed, or bored, you use food as a friend to make you feel better, you are, in essence, relying on food as an *emotional crutch* to support you in times of need.

How strongly can you relate to this?

How important is *eliminating* emotional eating? I firmly believe that unless you eliminate emotional eating, you will *never* truly reach your ultimate weight loss potential over the long term.

Imagine how effective you'd be if you could destroy this destructive behavior that has been sabotaging your weight loss. It's high time to learn how to achieve this.

By eliminating emotional eating from your life:

1. You *will no longer be a slave to food.*

2. Your weight loss *will become more consistent.*

3. Your 8 Minutes in the Morning plan will become *even easier for you to follow.*

What's my secret for eliminating emotional eating? I call it the Cruise Control™ Secret and it is made of up three simple steps:

Step 1. Identify the emotion that triggers you.

Step 2. Identify the opposite emotion.

Step 3. Create a new game plan.

Ready to start? Let's get to it!

STEP 1: Identify the Emotion That Triggers You

Identifying the specific primary emotion that triggers you to overeat is critical. Even though there might be several emotions that stimulate this response, there is only one primary destructive emotion that generates 80 percent or more of your emotional eating. This is the one we are going to focus on right now.

Before we begin, make sure you have a pen in hand. Once you are ready, close your eyes and imagine the last time you had a powerful emotional urge to overeat. How clearly can you see that happening? Envision it right now. Once you can vividly recall that moment, simply finish the following sentence by inserting the emotion that triggered you to overeat.

> ### "I feel the urge right now to use food to make me feel better because I am feeling _____."

EXAMPLES: Emptiness / Loneliness / Boredom / Depression / Stress / Anger / Guilt / Unworthiness

Still not sure what the emotion is that triggers you to overeat? Here are a couple of questions that might help you to define your emotional trigger:

1. When I know that I am overeating, what do I recall feeling just before I indulge?
2. What is the painful emotion that I feel most often in my life?

By writing down the primary emotion that triggers you to overeat, and seeing it on paper, you will establish *awareness* of this emotion. As it does for many of my clients, this recognition can cause such a "lightbulb" reaction that you will stop the emotional eating. Awareness is power. The quicker you acknowledge this trigger, the more successfully you will curb your emotional eating. But we are not done yet. Let's move on to the next step.

STEP 2: Identify the Opposite Emotion

This next step is very easy. Simply identify the emotion that is the exact opposite of the emotion in Step 1.

Why is this critical for your success? *This is the tool that will set you free from emotional eating.* This is the sensation that you are *desperately craving.* You are so severely dependent upon this emotion that up until now you have been willing to sacrifice your own health to attain it. Until now, food has been your primary source for its fulfillment. You can find a healthier way to improve your emotional well-being.

For example:

- If **emptiness** is your trigger to eat . . . then **LOVE** is what you have really been craving in your life. Bottom line: eating food has given you love.
- If **stress** is your trigger to eat . . . then **PEACEFULNESS** is what you have really been craving in your life. Bottom line: eating food has given you peace.
- If **boredom** is your trigger to eat . . . then **EXCITEMENT** is what you have really been craving in your life. Bottom line: eating food has given you excitement.
- If **loneliness** is your trigger to eat . . . then **CONNECTION** is what you have really been craving in your life. Bottom line: eating food has given you connection.
- If **anger** is your trigger to ea . . . then **HAPPINESS** is what you have really been craving in your life. Bottom line: eating food has given you happiness.

Does this make sense? Good. In the box below, simply write down the emotion that is the opposite of the emotion in step 1.

The emotion that is the opposite of the emotion in Step 1 is:

_____.

NOTE: Feeling this emotion (*without* using food) is the ticket to your freedom from emotional eating. We will do this in the next step.

EXAMPLES: Connection / Excitement / Relaxation / Joyfulness / Love / Peacefulness / Tranquility

STEP 3: Create a New Game Plan

The last step of the Cruise Control™ Secret is to create a new game plan that invokes more of this "opposite emotion" in your life, especially when you feel an emotional urge to eat when you are not hungry. Having the capability to harness this essential emotion without having to use food *will set you free*. The more you feel this *critical, positive emotion* on your own, the less you will wallow in your old destructive emotion, thereby removing the emotional urge to overeat. By filling yourself up with the emotion you *really* want, you will stop eating emotionally. It's that simple.

How do you create this new game plan?

All you need to do is ask yourself the following POWER QUESTION: "What would have to happen in order for me to feel more _____ in my life (without using food)?"

Now, on the line below, rewrite the emotion you wrote down in Step 2. This is your empowering emotion. Below it, I want you to ask the POWER QUESTION and come up with a list of 10 new things you enjoy that you can do anywhere—and that will provide you with this empowering feeling. Want some ideas? See the examples on the next page.

Got it? Great! Let's get the party started.

Your Game Plan Chart

THIS IS MY NEW GAME PLAN to feel more_____.

WRITE YOUR EMOTION FROM STEP 2 HERE.

Here are 10 things I can do on my own that will make me feel this essential emotion, but *without* eating.

1._____

2._____

3._____

4._____

5._____

6._____

7._____

8._____

9._____

10._____

NOTE: **Make three copies of this chart. Place one on your refrigerator. Carry one with you at all times. And give one to a friend who will hold you accountable.**

Game Plan Examples:

Jane's Empowering Emotion: LOVE

HER GAME PLAN:
1. Looking at photos of my family
2. Calling a close family member
3. Remembering a time when I felt love
4. Hugging my kids or husband
5. Playing with my puppy
6. Going out to lunch with my friends
7. Sending out cards with nice notes to my good friends
8. Enjoying my connection to God
9. Appreciating when people tell me they love me
10. Volunteering at a senior citizens center

Jan's Empowering Emotion: RELAXATION

HER GAME PLAN:
1. Getting a manicure
2. Watching TV
3. Sipping tea and reading a book
4. Indulging in a massage
5. Taking a walk on the beach
6. Meditating
7. Enjoying a day off from work
8. Going shopping
9. Painting
10. Soaking in a hot bath

Ann's Empowering Emotion: EXCITEMENT

HER GAME PLAN:
1. Participating in a dance class
2. Taking in painting or pottery lessons

3. Going to the movies once per week

4. Enjoying "date night" with my husband

5. Going to lunch with girlfriends once per week

6. Taking personal development seminars

7. Trying a new restaurant

8. Planning a vacation

9. Shopping

10. Reading or writing a book

FOR MORE EXAMPLES VISIT www.jorgecruise.com/cruisecontrol.

Bonus Tip

There's one essential activity that you should add to your game plan, no matter what. *Join our online support club.* In fact, the next time you feel your old debilitating emotion, instead of heading to the refrigerator, head to your computer. There, you can join the thousands of other 8 Minute Marvels at the JorgeCruise.com online community. Through contact with other people on the same weight loss path, you will gain a major support system.

How critical can the JorgeCruise.com online support group be to you? Well, meet one of my new 8 Minute Marvels (see photos in this section). What's Debra's weight loss secret? Of course she followed the 8 Minute program (read her success story), but she *also* became very actively involved in the 8 Minute online club at JorgeCruise.com. In fact, that is where I met her; it is where she shared her success story, and where she continues to thrive.

Weight loss research has shown very clearly that you are more likely to lose weight and keep it off for life when you do it with a support group. That's the power of an online club. And at JorgeCruise.com, it does not matter what city you live in, or what time of the day it is, or what you are wearing! Yep, you just need your computer and a connection to the Internet. It's that simple. So if you want a major support tool and resource, be sure to include "Become active at the JorgeCruise.com club" in your top ten game plan activities. I promise it will change your life and make your weight loss even easier and more fun.

Conclusion

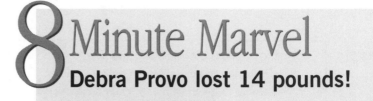

8 Minute Marvel
Debra Provo lost 14 pounds!

Well, you have done it! Congratulations. You now know my Cruise Control™ Secret for eliminating emotional eating. It will immediately transform your life!

Remember that emotional eating is the number one internal challenge that will continuously prevent you from achieving your ideal weight. Therefore, if you genuinely want to lose the weight, it is *essential* that you have access to a simple system that can immediately help you eliminate any emotional urge to overeat!

This is what I suggest you do right now. In addition to the chart I recommend you hang on your refrigerator, I'd like you to carry with you—everywhere you go for the next 28 days—a photocopy of your Cruise Control Game Plan chart. Anytime you

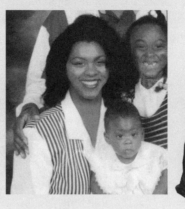

BEFORE

"Before 8 Minutes my blood pressure was 140/90, but now, since losing 14 pounds, it's around 108/68. What I love about the program is that the results of losing the weight are so quick and simple, and all you need is 8 Minutes in the Morning. Others in my family are trying the program. My mother-in-law has lost three pounds so far. And one of my sisters is now trying the program. So I am hopeful for many more success stories to come."

feel the urge to emotionally eat, I want you to immediately review it and begin one of your alternative activities.

And to give yourself a major advantage this very day, I recommend that you select one of the items from your list and indulge yourself in it within the next 60 minutes. Yes, *action is power*. And I want you to take action right now. Whatever you have to do . . . make it happen within 60 minutes of reading these words. I promise that by doing this, you will change your life! You will *no longer be a slave to food*, your weight loss *will become more consistent*, and your 8 Minutes in the Morning plan will become *even easier for you to follow*.

I know you will do great!

Good luck and best wishes,

Your coach—

JORGE

P.S. Once you have completed your positive alternative activity, I'd love for you to e-mail me at cruisecontrol@jorgecruise.com and let me know how the Cruise Control™ Secret has personally helped you to eliminate emotional eating from your life. Please let me know how your life has changed and share your game plan with me. I promise to write you back!

FOR MORE TIPS ON EMOTIONAL EATING FROM JORGE,
VISIT www.jorgecruise.com/cruisecontrol.

Become a Weight-Loss Star

Send Jorge Cruise your 8 Minutes in the Morning success story and you will qualify to have your story appear on Jorge Cruise's Web site! Your success story could be seen by millions of people. It will not only acknowledge your hard work but also help inspire others to improve their lives. Get ready to step up and become part of Jorge's weight-loss revolution!

Here's what to do.

1. Write your story (of at least 150 words), sharing your 8 Minutes in the Morning weight-loss transformation. Describe what your life was like before you started the program and what your life is like now. Include your height, starting weight, your new weight, and how long it took you to arrive at your goal weight.

2. Include a full-body "before" and "after" photo. Make sure your "after" photo is a recent picture. Send either prints or scanned photographs.

3. E-mail your story and photos to stories@jorgecruise.com or find the post office address at www.jorgecruise.com/mail. Be sure to include your name, address, phone number, and e-mail address.

As a thank-you for sending in your letter and photos, you will automatically be entered into Jorge's monthly success-story drawing. Each month, Jorge personally selects one lucky Weight-Loss Star to receive a free personal phone-coaching session with him (a $200 value). If you are selected, you will hear directly from Jorge! And if you submit your photos and success story via e-mail, you will also receive a special e-mail from Jorge with advanced tips on how to take your 8 Minutes in the Morning workout to the next level.

Good luck and best wishes!

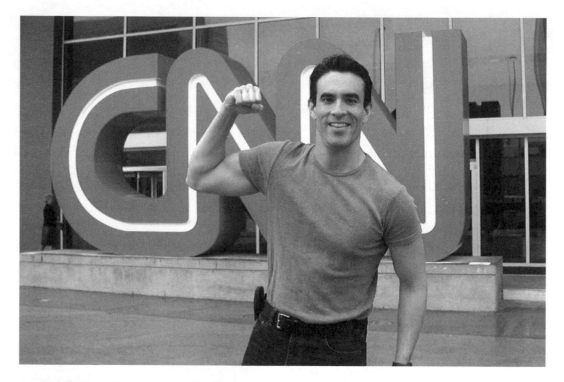

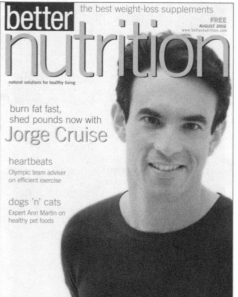

"America's newest weight-loss guru!"

—*Better Nutrition* magazine

About Jorge Cruise:
America's #1 Online Weight-Loss Specialist

Jorge Cruise is the *New York Times* **bestselling weight-loss author** of *8 Minutes in the Morning* and is recognized as the **number one online weight-loss specialist**, due to his unprecedented success in helping more than 3 million time-deprived people lose weight at www.jorgecruise.com

Jorge has been featured in the *New York Times, USA Today, People, Woman's World, First for Women, Prevention, Self, FIT*, and has appeared on *Oprah*, CNN, *Good Morning America*, and Lifetime.

No other trainer has had so many people directly reveal what really works in getting fast and lasting weight-loss results. This makes Jorge one of the most up-to-date and in-demand trainers both online and off-line.

Jorge is a nominee for Fitness Instructor of the year by IDEA, the national association of fitness professionals and was named by Arnold Schwarzenegger as a special advisor to the California Governor's Council on Physical Fitness and Sports.

In addition, **Jorge is a journalist** for various television shows and magazines such as *First for Women, Prevention* magazine, ABC television and Univision. He is a member of the Association of Health Care Journalists, a nonprofit organization dedicated to advancing public understanding of health care issues. He is fluent in both English and Spanish.

Utilizing the knowledge and credentials that he has gained from the University of California, San Diego (UCSD), Dartmouth College, the Cooper Institute for Aerobics Research, the American College of Sports Medicine (ACSM), and the American Council on Exercise (ACE), Jorge is dedicated to helping time deprived women, men, kids, and seniors lose weight *and achieve their dreams!*

Photo Credits

Front cover photo © Robert Trachtenberg

Back cover photos courtesy of Jorge Cruise, Inc.

Interior photos by Mitch Mandel/Rodale Images, except the following:

Robert Trachtenberg: pp. 12, 199

Courtesy of Jorge Cruise, Inc.: pp. xiii, xv, 4, 6, 7, 9, 16, 17, 39, 41, 42, 47, 60, 106, 107, 135,163, 191, 193, 196, 246

Courtesy of Rodale Images: pp. 64, 67

Better Nutrition magazine/Sabot Publishing: p. 246

First for Women issue #18, May 6, 2002: p. 182

Index

Underscored page references indicate boxed text.

Bagels, 156
Basil as salt substitute, 192
Beans
  as protein source, 60
  recipes
    Burrito, 230
    Three-Bean Salad, 229
Bedtime, changing, 45
Behavior change
  asking the Master Question, 150
  dissatisfaction as tool for, 86
  reclaiming wasted time, 102
  replacing bad habits with good, 126
  through Result-Driven Questions, 98
Biceps exercises
  hammer, 119
  one-arm curl, 147
  seated curl, 147
  standing curl, 91
Biology of Success, 134
Blood pressure, morning exercise and, 45
Blood sugar regulation
  complex carbohydrates and, 61–62
  omega fats for, 54
Body image
  designing your body, 82
  visualizing your dream body, 94
Body measurements, 23
Body movement
  mood and, 122
  music and, 138
Books on weight loss, 186, 188
Boredom, eating and, 238
Bread, whole grain, 168
Breathing, deep
  for energy and mood, 142
  exercises for, 142
  to prevent cravings, 68
Broccoli
  Asian Broccoli and Cauliflower Salad, 227
  for calcium, 64
Butter, olive oil as substitute, 55, 128
Butters, nut, 124
Butt exercises
  kickup, 99
  leg lift, 155
  squeeze, 127
  wide squeeze, 183

C

Caffeine
  cravings and, 72
  sleep disruption and, 45
  thirst due to, 72
Calcium, nondairy sources of, 64
Calf exercises
  seated raise, 127, 183
  standing heel raise, 99, 155
Calories
  in fruit juices, 72, 73
  in fruits, 67
  intake, in the Eating Card System, 71, 211
  from nibbling and snacking, 100
  powerwalking and, 199–200
  in vegetables, 65
Cancer
  as obesity-related illness, 13
  omega fats and, 54
  soy and, 61
Canola oil, 56
Carbohydrates
  complex
    breads, whole grain, 168
    insulin levels and, 61, 168
    portions, in the Eating Card System, 213–14
    role in fat loss, 61–62
    vs. simple carbohydrates, 62
  simple
    body fat and, 62
    insulin levels and, 61
    vs. complex carbohydrates, 62
Casein, 64, 132
Cauliflower
  Asian Broccoli and Cauliflower Salad, 227
Celery, as healthy snack, 148
Cell membrane health, omega fats for, 52, 55–57
Cereals, breakfast, 63
Cheerios, 63
Cheese
  pizza without, 104
  soy cheese as substitute, 64, 132
Chest exercises
  dumbbell press, 83
  fly, 139
  knee pushup, 111
  pushup, 167

E

Eating Card System
  adjusting, after weight loss, 195
  cards to photocopy, 234
  dietary fat and, 58–59
  how it works, 69–70, 233
  as part of daily program, 79
  portion size tips, 59
  protein intake and, 60
  reference guide to foods, 211–18
    alcohol, 217
    complex carbohydrates, 213–14
    dairy foods, 214
    fast foods, 217–18
    fat, 211
    fruits, 216
    protein, 212–13
    treats and cravings, 216–17
    vegetables, 215
Eating out tips, 72, 160
Eating Well for Optimal Health, 64
Egg whites
  Egg-White Scramble, 229
  as protein source, 60
Emotional fitness. *See also* Internal transformation
    exercises
  committing yourself to success, 27–29
  deciding what you want, 22–27
  emotional eating
    game plan for, 238–43
    identifying emotions, 236–38
    Jorge's Web site, 243
    steps to eliminate, 235–41
  as foundation for program, 16
  journal keeping and, 20–21
  as program component, 10
  success story, 17–18
  taking internal control, 18–19
  Wake-Up Talks and, 19–20
Emptiness, emotional eating and, 238
Endorphins and exercise, 44–45, 46
Equipment needed for program, 37–38
Essential fatty acids. *See* Omega fats
Exercise. *See also* Exercises; Strength training
  aerobic
    cardiovascular system health and, 14
    difficulty of, if obese, 14, 35, 200–201
    metabolism not increased, 37

    not for weight loss, 14
    powerwalking, 199–204
  as part of daily program, 77, 79
  powerwalking, 199–204
  self-consciousness and, 202
  Tai chi, 195
  Web sites about, 178
  yoga, 195
Exercises (Today's Moves)
  for abdominals
    crunch, 87, 143
    lower pull, 115, 171
  for arms
    dip (triceps), 119
    hammer (biceps), 119
    lying kickback (triceps), 91
    one-arm curl (biceps), 147
    seated curl (biceps), 175
    seated overhead (triceps), 175
    standing curl (biceps), 91
    standing kickback (triceps), 147
  for back
    bird dog, 111
    standing bent-over row, 139
    superman, 167
    two-arm row, 83
  for butt
    kickup, 99
    leg lift, 155
    squeeze, 127
    wide squeeze, 183
  for chest
    dumbbell press, 83
    fly, 139
    knee pushup, 111
    pushup, 167
  for legs
    doggie (outer thigh), 103
    frog (inner thigh), 131
    hamstring leg lift, 95, 179
    inner-thigh leg raise, 103, 187
    leg curl (hamstrings), 123
    leg raise (outer thigh), 131, 187
    lunge (quadriceps), 123
    one-leg curl (hamstrings), 151
    pep leader (outer thigh), 159
    plie (inner thigh), 159
    seated raise (calves), 127, 183
    squat (quadriceps), 95
    standing heel raise (calves), 99, 155

standing raise (quadriceps), 151
the wall (quadriceps), 179
for shoulders
bent-over lateral raise, 143
forward raise, 171
lateral raise, 87
overhead press, 115

F

Family success story, 39
Fast food portions, in the Eating Card System, 217–18
Fat, body. *See also* Obesity
brown fat vs. white fat, 52–53
carbohydrates and, 61–62
lack of dietary protein and, 59
omega fats and, 52–53
Fat, dietary, *See also specific types*
as appetite suppressant, 48, 51
bad
addictive nature of, 50
effect of, on body, 53
heat-processed, 50
saturated fats, 49, 144
trans fats, 49, 50
to boost metabolism, 48
Eating Card System and, 58–59
home experiment with fat types, 54
misunderstandings about, 48–49
omega fats
3 types recommended, 50
to boost metabolism, 52
percentage of, in oils (chart), 56
role in body, 50
to unlock stored body fat, 48
portions, in the Eating Card System, 211
Fat-free diets, 48–49
Fatigue, dehydration and, 69
Fiber
vegetables and, 65
whole grains and, 63
Fish
marinade for, 120
as protein source, 60
recipes
Salmon Salad, 231
Tuna Melt, 230

salad, healthy, 152
tips for adding to diet, 120
Flax for Life, 51
Flax oil
importance of, in weight loss, 57–58
percentage of omega fats in (chart), 56
as source of Omega 3, 51
tips for adding to diet, 58
Flu, garlic for, 184
Food. *See also* Eating out
emotional eating, 235–41
portions determination, 59, 211–18
when intertwined with love, 4–5
Foods, *See also specific names of oils. See also* Nutrition;
Recipes; Snacking
almond butter, 124
bagels, 156
bread, whole grain, 168
chocolate, 68, 136
dairy, 64, 128, 132, 214
fish, 60, 120, 152
fruit juices, 92
fruit, limiting in diet, 66–67, 68
grapes, frozen, 108
low-fat, obesity and, 62
peanut butter, 124
reference guide to, 211–18
sweet, insulin and, 52
Treats and Cravings foods, 67–68
vegetables, 65–66, 112, 116, 140
Fruit
advice for fruit lovers, 68
juices
best choices, 73
calories in, 72, 92
diluting, with sparkling water, 92
limiting, in diet, 66–67
portions, in the Eating Card System, 216

G

Garlic
for immune system, 184
as vegetable seasoning, 116
Germany, obesity in, 13
Glucagon
carbohydrates and, 61–62
fruit and, 67

Ready for more?

Check out these ways to take 8 Minutes in the Morning *to the next level.*

■ Online Support: Jorgecruise.com
The #1 Weight-Loss club for Busy People

To be truly successful at weight loss you must also connect with others. Trying to lose weight alone is a formula for failure. The need to talk with others who are also losing weight is very important. This need to connect is sometimes even more important than the need to lose weight. Bottom line, you must get encouragement and support. Weight loss desires company and the ALL-NEW www.JorgeCruise.com will provide you with the undying support you require.

- Daily messages from Jorge
- Weekly online meetings
- Live chat auditoriums with Jorge
- Expert advice from 8 Minutes mentors
- Chart your weight loss
- And much more . . .

Joining Jorge's ALL-NEW online weight-loss club *is like joining a family!*

■ The Exercise Video

Personally experience Jorge Cruise's dynamic coaching style in your own home!

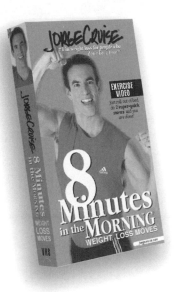

With this high-energy video, you will feel that you are shoulder-to-shoulder with your weight-loss coach, Jorge Cruise. He will walk you through, step-by-step, one week's worth of his superquick *8 Minutes in the Morning*™ weight-loss moves. It could not be easier.

- The ideal companion to your book
- No special exercise equipment required
- Motivating and energetic music that makes it more fun

■ The Weight-Loss Supplement

Bring back the joy of eating with Jorge Cruise's all-natural Flax Oil Complex

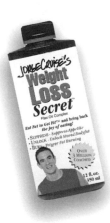

Jorge Cruise's *Weight Loss Secret*™ is an all-natural flax oil complex that helps control your hunger and tastes great on food. Flax oil contains the very beneficial omega-3 fats that are critical to successful weight loss and long-term health.

- Satisfies your hunger so you will not overeat
- Includes the natural fat-burning enzyme Lipase
- All natural—absolutely no stimulants

ON-THE-GO WEIGHT LOSS TRAVEL CARDS

EQUIPMENT: You will need one set of dumbbells; the weight you select should be challenging by the 12th repetition. (If you can easily complete 12 repetitions, the weight is not sufficient.)

PROGRAM: Begin with a quick warm-up. Follow with one set of 12 repetitions from the first of the day's exercises, then immediately do one set of 12 reps from the second exercise. Repeat the cycle for a total of four sets of each exercise.

Monday

Dumbbell Press (Chest): Lie on your back with knees bent and feet flat on the floor. Use a pillow under your back and head for support if desired. Hold a dumbbell in each hand, line up elbows with shoulders, bend arms to right angles. Exhale as you extend your arms toward the ceiling. Hold for 1 second. Inhale as you lower arms.

EXERCISE A

Tuesday

Lateral Raise (Shoulders): Stand with your feet shoulder-width apart, back straight. Hold a dumbbell in each hand, arms straight at your sides, elbows slightly bent. Exhale as you lift the dumbbells out to the side, stopping slightly above shoulder level, palms facing the floor. Hold for 1 second. Inhale as you lower.

EXERCISE A

Wednesday

Lying Kickback (Triceps): Lie on a mat with knees bent and feet flat on the floor. Hold a dumbbell in each hand by your ears, elbows pointing up. Exhale as you raise the dumbbells toward the ceiling. Hold for 1 second. Inhale as you lower.

EXERCISE A

Thursday

Leg Lift (Hamstrings): Lie on a mat with palms flat on the floor and heels on the seat of a sturdy chair. Exhale as you contract the backs of your thighs to push your butt toward the ceiling. Hold for 1 second. Inhale as you slowly lower.

EXERCISE A

Friday

Standing Heel Raise (Calves): Stand with feet shoulder-width apart. Hold a dumbbell in each hand, arms at your sides. Keep your chest out, shoulder blades rolled back and down. Exhale as you lift heels and rise onto tiptoes. Hold for 1 second. Inhale as you lower.

EXERCISE A

Saturday **Leg Raise (Inner Thigh):**

Lie on a mat on your left side with left elbow supporting upper body, left leg extended. Bend right knee and place your right foot behind your left leg for balance. Keeping left leg straight, exhale as you lift the foot as high as you can. Hold for 1 second. Inhale as you lower. Do one set with your left leg, then switch sides.

EXERCISE A

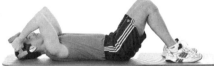
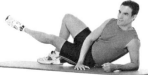
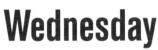
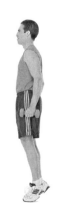

ON-THE-GO WEIGHT LOSS TRAVEL CARDS

Tuesday

Crunch (Abdominals): Lie on a mat on your back with knees bent and feet flat on the floor. To prevent neck strain, make a fist with one hand and place it between your chin and collarbone. Grasp wrist with other hand. Exhale and slowly curl your upper torso until your shoulder blades are off the ground. Hold for 1 second. Inhale as you lower.

EXERCISE B

www.jorgecruise.com

Monday

Two-Arm Row (Back): While seated, grasp a dumbbell in each hand. Use a pillow on your lap for support if desired. Lean forward, extend arms straight down, elbows slightly bent. Exhale as you bend your elbows and bring them toward the ceiling, stopping when hands are parallel to the thighs. Hold for 1 second. Inhale as you lower.

EXERCISE B

www.jorgecruise.com

Thursday

Squat (Quadriceps): Stand with feet slightly wider than shoulder-width apart and arms at your sides. Keeping your back straight, exhale as you squat down to about 90 degrees, pushing your butt out as if you were sitting into a chair. Don't let your knees extend forward past your toes. Hold for 1 second. Inhale as you straighten legs.

EXERCISE B

www.jorgecruise.com

Wednesday

Standing Curl (Biceps): Stand with feet shoulder-width apart and arms extended by your sides. Hold a dumbbell in each hand, palms facing forward. Exhale and curl both arms to just past 90 degrees, keeping your elbows at your sides. Hold for 1 second. Inhale as you lower.

EXERCISE B

www.jorgecruise.com

Saturday **Doggie (Outer Thigh):**

Kneel on a mat on all fours with knees hip-width apart, hands placed slightly wider than your shoulders, and fingers pointing forward. Keep your back straight and head up. Exhale as you raise your right leg, bent at a 90-degree angle. Hold for 1 second. Inhale as you lower. Do one set with your right leg, then switch sides.

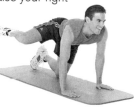

EXERCISE B

www.jorgecruise.com

Friday **Kickup (Butt):**

Kneel on a mat on all fours with knees hip-width apart, hands slightly wider than your shoulders, fingers pointing forward. Keeping your head up, raise your left leg until your thigh is in line with your torso. Bend your knee and exhale as you push your foot toward the ceiling. Once you've reached your maximum contraction, hold for 1 second. Inhale as you lower. Do one set with your left leg, then switch sides.

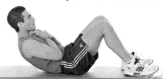

EXERCISE B

www.jorgecruise.com